# DOOMSCROLL
# DETOX

**Alvin Mercer** is a digital wellness strategist and former behavioural design consultant who spent over a decade helping tech companies craft addictive user experiences—before switching sides. Now, he writes and speaks about reclaiming attention, resisting manipulation, and building healthier relationships with technology. With a background in cognitive psychology and UX design, Mercer brings insider clarity to the dark art of digital distraction. *Doomscroll Detox* is his urgent, no-nonsense guide for breaking the cycle and reclaiming your mind. Alvin splits his time between Berlin and Brooklyn, where he runs retreats on digital minimalism and occasionally turns his phone off for entire weekends.

# DOOMSCROLL
# DETOX

### RECLAIMING YOUR BRAIN
### IN THE AGE OF CLICKBAIT

## ALVIN MERCER

RUPA

Published by
Rupa Publications India Pvt. Ltd 2025
161-B/4, Gulmohar House,
Yusuf Sarai Community Centre,
New Delhi 110049

*Sales centres:*
Bengaluru Chennai
Hyderabad Kolkata Mumbai

Edition Copyright © Rupa Publications India Pvt. Ltd 2025

The views and opinions expressed in this book are the
author's own and the facts are as reported by him which
have been verified to the extent possible, and the publishers
are not in any way liable for the same.

P-ISBN: 978-93-7003-236-1
E-ISBN: 978-93-7003-027-5

First impression 2025

10 9 8 7 6 5 4 3 2 1

The moral right of the author has been asserted

Printed in India

# Contents

## Part 3: Why It's So Hard to Stop

## Part 4: Reclaiming Your Mind (Without Quitting the Internet)

## Part 5: Building a Healthier Digital Future

PART 1

# Hooked & Hijacked – How the Internet Took Over

# 1

# Why You Can't Look Away

THERE'S A REASON YOUR THUMB moves before your brain even registers it. The moment your screen lights up, it's almost automatic—open, scroll, refresh. Maybe you meant to check one thing. Maybe you told yourself it'd be quick. But then one post turns into ten, ten turns into fifty, and suddenly, you're knee-deep in a stranger's vacation photos, a Twitter thread about drama that doesn't concern you, and a TikTok rabbit hole that started with cute dogs and somehow led to conspiracy theories. You don't even know how you got here. You just know you can't stop.

This isn't just bad self-control. It's design.

Social media isn't just a tool—it's an ecosystem built to keep you glued. Platforms aren't hoping you'll spend time there— they're making sure you do. Every swipe, every refresh, every little hit of novelty is a carefully curated dopamine loop, engineered to keep your brain on the hook. The question isn't why you can't stop scrolling—it's how anyone ever does. Before the digital age, information had an endpoint. Books had final pages. Newspapers got tossed. TV shows rolled credits. But now? There is no end. Your feed isn't a timeline; it's an infinity pool—bottomless, endless, designed so that the moment you consume, there's more waiting for you.

That "pull-to-refresh" motion? It's not just functional—it's psychological conditioning. It mimics the mechanics of a slot machine. You swipe down, and maybe you get something exciting, maybe you don't. Either way, you keep pulling. It's a game of endless rewards, one that your brain is wired to play.

And autoplay? Even worse. You were going to stop at one video, but before your brain can even process that intention, the next clip starts rolling. Now your decision isn't whether to watch—it's whether to interrupt something already in motion. And just like that, you're stuck in the loop.

## Your Brain on Scroll Mode: Why It Feels So Good (And So Bad)

Ever notice how time disappears when you're deep in your feed? That's because scrolling puts you in a low-effort, high-reward state. Your brain doesn't have to work—it just has to receive. And every new post, video, or meme is a tiny hit of dopamine, the neurotransmitter that fuels pleasure and motivation.

Dopamine loves novelty. It thrives on the unexpected. That's why social media isn't just entertaining—it's addictive. Your brain gets a reward for every new piece of content, reinforcing the behavior. The more you scroll, the more your brain craves more scrolling. But here's the kicker: dopamine spikes aren't the same as real satisfaction. That quick hit of pleasure doesn't last, which is why the second you stop scrolling, you don't feel good—you feel drained, foggy, maybe even guilty. Because scrolling isn't just taking up time. It's rewiring your brain to need constant stimulation.

Ever wonder why focusing on a book or even a long article feels harder than it used to? That's not just attention span decay—that's your brain adjusting to a world of instant, rapid-fire content. You've been conditioned to consume fast, shallow, and endlessly.

And deep thinking? It doesn't stand a chance.

## You're Not Addicted—You're Hooked (And There's a Difference)

There's a common misconception that people are addicted to their phones. But the truth? Most of us aren't addicted to the device itself. We're hooked on the way it delivers content. We don't compulsively check our phones because we love the hardware— we check them because they're the portal to the next hit of engagement, information, or entertainment. The reason it's so hard to stop isn't because of lack of willpower. It's because the system is built to make quitting feel uncomfortable, unnatural, and even anxiety-inducing.

Ever feel that weird sense of unease when you don't check your phone? That's not an accident. The constant exposure to micro-rewards (likes, notifications, new posts) keeps your brain in a state of expectation. Your mind starts to anticipate the next reward before it even happens. And when you don't get it? Your brain panics. It nudges you—go check, just in case.

And if you resist? You might feel like you're missing out, like something important is happening without you. That's not FOMO in the traditional sense—it's a dopamine withdrawal symptom.

If this all sounds bleak—good news. Just like your brain **adapted** to infinite scrolling, it can **un-adapt**, too. But the key isn't quitting cold turkey or deleting every app (because let's be real, you're not about to do that). The key is to **recognize the mechanics** at play and disrupt them just enough to break the trance.

Here's how:

Pause before you refresh. Just a three-second delay before opening an app can snap you out of autopilot. Ask yourself: Do

I actually want to check this, or am I just programmed to?

Interrupt the loop. Mid-scroll, stop and look around. Take a breath. Just a moment of mindfulness can break the unconscious cycle.

Turn off autoplay. This one's non-negotiable. Make content consumption a choice, not a reflex.

Switch "pull-to-refresh" with actual movement. Every time you feel the urge, stand up, stretch, or do something physical. Give your brain a different dopamine hit—one that doesn't involve endless scrolling.

Most importantly? Remember that the urge to scroll isn't about self-control—it's about conditioning. You're not weak for getting caught in the loop. You're **human**. And in an era where everything is engineered to steal your attention, learning to **take it back** might just be the ultimate power move.

# 2

# How Your Brain Got Hacked

PICTURE THIS—YOU POST A PHOTO. Maybe it's a spontaneous selfie or the kind of carefully curated shot you spent twenty minutes perfecting. Either way, you hit "share" and wait. A like pops up. Then another. A comment rolls in. And whether you admit it or not, there's a tiny spark—an electric little buzz that feels good. Really good. It's almost subconscious, that rush of satisfaction. But it's not random. It's chemical. And it's exactly why platforms have you right where they want you.

At the core of it all is dopamine—your brain's reward currency. It's the neurotransmitter responsible for those fleeting moments of pleasure and motivation. Dopamine is why that first sip of coffee feels like a warm hug to your soul. It's why you crave a text back from your crush. And in the digital age, it's why you can lose hours of your day scrolling through strangers' lives while your to-do list collects dust. Because social media isn't just giving you content—it's serving up dopamine hits on demand, and your brain can't resist the pull.

The scary part? It's not even an accident. Social platforms are engineered to tap into your brain's most primal reward system. The algorithms behind them don't just work with your habits—they shape them. And every like, comment, and notification is part of a bigger design that hijacks your brain's chemistry. Once you understand how it works, it becomes impossible to unsee—and much harder to keep pretending you're in control.

## When Social Media Feels Like a Slot Machine

There's a reason you reach for your phone the second you feel bored—or sad, or anxious, or even just vaguely restless. The pull isn't just about distraction—it's about the possibility of reward. And the way social media keeps those rewards unpredictable? That's not a glitch. It's the same mechanism that makes gambling so addictive.

It's called variable reinforcement, and it's pure psychological magic. When you open an app, you never know what you're going to get—maybe it's a flood of likes, or maybe it's nothing. That uncertainty is the hook. If you knew exactly how many likes a post would get, you'd lose interest. But when the outcome is unpredictable, your brain stays engaged, chasing the next possible reward. Every time you swipe, scroll, or refresh, it's like pulling the lever on a slot machine—and once you're in that loop, it's hard to break free.

The most insidious part? Social media platforms know this and use it to their advantage. Instagram doesn't always show likes in real-time—they batch them together to deliver a bigger dopamine hit. TikTok's "For You" page is a masterclass in variable reinforcement, serving up an endless stream of videos tailored to your every subconscious craving. And when notifications are delayed just enough to keep you wondering, your brain stays on high alert, waiting for the next dose of validation.

You're not scrolling because you're bored. You're scrolling because your brain has learned that somewhere in that endless feed, a reward is waiting—and it's been trained not to stop until it finds one.

## The Highs Are Cheap—And the Lows Hit Harder

Dopamine isn't inherently bad. It's the reason you feel joy when you accomplish something meaningful. It fuels motivation, focus, and pleasure. But not all dopamine is created equal. The kind you get from real-world experiences—connecting with a friend, achieving a goal, or even enjoying a sunset—comes with depth. It lingers. It satisfies.

But the dopamine you get from social media? It's a cheap thrill—fast, fleeting, and ultimately hollow. And over time, the constant flood of digital stimulation messes with your brain's natural reward system. You become less sensitive to everyday joys and more dependent on the quick, artificial hits that platforms provide.

Ever noticed how nothing feels as satisfying as that one viral post or those notifications lighting up your lock screen? That's not a coincidence. Your baseline for happiness shifts. What used to feel fulfilling—like a long conversation or finishing a project—starts to feel dull in comparison to the instant gratification your phone provides. And the more you chase those quick hits, the harder it becomes to find joy in the things that actually matter.

It's no wonder that anxiety and depression have skyrocketed in the age of social media. When your brain is wired for constant stimulation, stillness feels unbearable. When your self-worth is tied to digital approval, real-life connection feels fragile. And when every moment is interrupted by a screen, it's easy to lose touch with what you actually want—because you're too busy chasing what the algorithm tells you to want.

## Your Brain Is Not Broken—It's Overstimulated

It's easy to feel like the problem is you—like you're weak for checking your phone mid-conversation or wasting hours on content you barely care about. But the truth? You're not broken. You're overstimulated. Your brain isn't designed for the relentless flood of information that modern technology provides. And when you're exposed to constant dopamine spikes, your natural reward pathways become overloaded.

In a way, it's like living in a world where dessert is always within arm's reach. At first, it's thrilling. But eventually, the sugar highs wear off faster, and you need more to feel satisfied. And real food—the nourishing stuff—starts to lose its appeal. That's what digital dopamine does. It trains your brain to seek out the quickest, easiest rewards, even if they leave you feeling empty afterward.

And the consequences? They're not just emotional—they're neurological. Studies show that excessive screen time physically reshapes parts of your brain responsible for focus, memory, and emotional regulation. It's no coincidence that attention spans are shrinking while burnout is rising. When your brain is trapped in a constant cycle of stimulation and depletion, it's harder to focus, harder to rest, and much harder to feel genuinely fulfilled.

## Taking Back Control

The good news? Your brain is adaptable. Just as it's been trained to crave the constant buzz of digital life, it can be retrained to find joy in slower, deeper experiences. But breaking the dopamine loop isn't about self-control—it's about reclaiming your attention from systems that are built to hijack it.

And here's the thing: You don't need to quit the internet to do it. You just need to interrupt the pattern. Small changes—like delaying your first scroll of the day, muting non-essential notifications, or creating phone-free zones—can start to reset your brain's reward system. When you give yourself space to breathe between dopamine hits, you start to rediscover the quieter pleasures—ones that no algorithm can manufacture.

Most importantly, recognize this: the problem was never you. You're not weak for getting hooked. You're living in a world designed to make you crave more, chase more, need more. And realizing that? It's the first step toward wanting less.

# 3

# The Algorithm Puppeteer

EVER WONDER WHY YOUR FEED feels like it *knows* you—sometimes better than you know yourself? That eerie sense that the internet is reading your mind isn't a coincidence. It's the work of algorithms—silent, invisible forces that shape everything you see, click, and crave. Behind every scroll, like, and tap is a meticulously crafted system designed not just to reflect your interests but to **mold them**. And while you might feel like you're in control, the truth is, you're not the one pulling the strings.

Algorithms—the invisible puppeteers of your online experience—are more than just lines of code. They're powerful prediction machines fueled by your every digital move. Every time you pause on a post, click a link, or linger a second longer on a video, you're feeding the algorithm. And in return, it feeds you back—content chosen to keep your attention locked in place. This isn't just about convenience; it's about **control**. The more an algorithm understands you, the easier it becomes to keep you hooked. And the longer you stay, the more valuable you are. Because in the attention economy, **your focus is currency**—and algorithms are programmed to make sure you never stop spending it.

It's easy to think your feed is a reflection of your choices. You follow who you want, like what you like, and the rest just falls into place. Except, that's not how it works. What you see online isn't random—it's **curated**. And the algorithm's job isn't to show you everything—it's to show you **what will keep you watching**.

At their core, social media algorithms are prediction engines. They analyze **patterns of behavior**—not just what you do, but how long you do it. Did you pause on a video? Watch it twice? Share it with a friend? Each interaction feeds the machine, helping it refine what to show you next. And because these systems are designed to maximize engagement, they prioritize content that triggers **strong reactions**—whether it's excitement, outrage, or envy.

It's why your feed isn't filled with the most balanced, thoughtful content—it's filled with **what makes you feel the most**. The algorithm doesn't care if that viral post makes you laugh or leaves you spiraling in existential dread. All that matters is that it keeps you **scrolling**. And the longer you stay, the more data you give—and the smarter the algorithm becomes.

The most unsettling part? These systems don't just track what you **explicitly** engage with. They observe everything—from the milliseconds you hover over an image to the videos you almost watched but didn't. Even your moments of hesitation become **data points**, shaping the next wave of content designed to capture your attention.

And once the algorithm knows what you want—sometimes before you do—it stops being a mirror of your preferences and starts **shaping them**. It decides which voices you hear, which stories matter, and what realities you believe in. It's not just showing you the world—it's **building one around you**.

## When the Algorithm Knows You Better Than You Know Yourself

Algorithms aren't just tracking your interests—they're **predicting your next move**. Behind the scenes, advanced AI systems analyze millions of data points to create an eerily accurate profile of who you are. Every purchase, search query, and late-night scroll paints a more vivid picture. And these systems don't just know what you like—they know **why you like it**, and they use that knowledge to guide your future choices.

Imagine an algorithm that knows you're about to burn out before you do—because it's seen your late-night doomscrolling spike, your increased searches for "how to be productive," and the way you've been clicking on motivational quotes. Now, your feed subtly shifts. Suddenly, you're drowning in ads for wellness retreats, productivity hacks, and "life-changing" apps. It feels like the universe is speaking directly to you—but really, it's the algorithm **nudging** you toward whatever keeps you on the hook.

And it doesn't stop at your phone. Algorithms track your location, your spending habits, even your **emotional rhythms**. Ever wonder why you suddenly crave a new outfit after scrolling through a breakup meme? That's the algorithm, working in real-time to **anticipate your desires**. And with every click, it gets better at guessing what you'll want next.

These predictive systems are so advanced, they can even detect **when you're vulnerable**—and they exploit those moments. If you've ever felt like your phone *knows* when you're lonely, anxious, or bored, that's not intuition—it's data. The algorithm watches for patterns in your behavior and delivers content tailored to keep you distracted, comforted, or spending. And the scariest part? You don't even realize it's happening.

## Are You Being Nudged—Or Manipulated?

The lines between **suggestion** and **manipulation** are blurrier than ever. When an algorithm "nudges" you, it's using subtle cues to influence your decisions. It's why a recommendation feels so personal—because it is. But those nudges aren't always innocent. They're designed to shape your behavior in ways that benefit the platform—**not you**.

Consider how quickly social media can shift your beliefs. You click on one conspiracy-adjacent video, and suddenly your feed is flooded with similar content. Not because it's true—but because it's **engaging**. Algorithms don't have ethics; they have goals. And if outrage and misinformation get more clicks than truth and nuance, guess which one wins?

And the influence doesn't stop at what you watch—it extends to **what you buy**, **who you trust**, and **how you see yourself**. Fashion trends, beauty standards, even your sense of identity— algorithms amplify what's profitable, often at the expense of what's real. You think you're making independent choices, but in reality? You're being **steered**.

## Taking Back the Strings

Here's the truth: You can't fully escape the algorithm's reach—but you **can** reclaim some control. It starts with recognizing when you're being **nudged**. That impulse to check your phone first thing in the morning? Not random. That sudden urge to buy something because "everyone else has it"? Manufactured. The key is to pause long enough to **question** the impulse.

Start by disrupting the algorithm's grip on your attention. Diversify your information sources—step outside the curated echo chamber. Take back your browsing habits by turning off autoplay, muting hyper-targeted ads, and opting out of endless recommendations. And most importantly, reclaim your **time**. The less you engage mindlessly, the harder it becomes for the algorithm to map your every move.

Remember, the algorithm isn't inherently evil—it's just **hungry**. It thrives on your clicks, your curiosity, your endless attention. But you don't have to give it everything. In a world where invisible systems are designed to pull your strings, the greatest rebellion is to cut the cords—and choose for **yourself**.

# 4

# Your Attention Is for Sale

IF YOU'VE EVER FELT LIKE the internet is competing for your focus—it is. Every notification, pop-up, and viral post isn't just there for your entertainment. It's there because your attention is the most **profitable** thing you possess. Behind the endless stream of content lies a multi-billion-dollar industry where your time is the product and your focus fuels the machine. But this isn't just a casual trade—you're part of a system meticulously designed to **capture and sell** your attention to the highest bidder.

Think about it. Every time you stop to check a post, watch a video, or scroll through a feed, you're contributing to a vast, invisible marketplace. But instead of exchanging money, you're offering up your most precious resource—**your time**. And in a world where people are constantly online, that time is as good as gold. Social media platforms, streaming services, and search engines aren't providing free content out of generosity—they're doing it because the longer they hold your attention, the more **valuable** you become. Your focus isn't just a side effect of modern technology—it's the **commodity** being bought and sold.

## The Business of Keeping You Hooked

At the heart of this system is a simple truth: **engagement equals profit**. The more time you spend on a platform, the more data you generate. And that data—your habits, preferences, and even your moods—becomes the raw material for an entire economy built around **predicting and influencing** your behavior. The longer you linger, the more advertisers are willing to pay to reach you. And platforms will do almost anything to keep you there.

It's why your feed is an endless buffet of hyper-personalized content. Every interaction you make is logged, analyzed, and used to shape what you see next. Did you watch a makeup tutorial all the way through? Expect a flood of beauty ads. Spent too long on a travel vlog? Suddenly, your feed is filled with dreamy vacation deals. This isn't coincidence—it's **intentional engineering**. Platforms don't just observe what you like—they push you toward **what they can sell**.

What makes this system so powerful is that it doesn't need you to **buy** something immediately. All it needs is your attention. Because in the attention economy, **time is the real transaction**. Every second you spend online translates into revenue—whether it's through direct ad clicks or the subtle shaping of future purchases. You aren't just a user; you're a **data point** in a vast commercial ecosystem where your focus is the ultimate prize.

And the tactics used to hold your attention are far from accidental. Infinite scrolling, autoplay videos, and curated feeds are carefully designed to **reduce friction**—the less effort it takes to stay, the harder it is to leave. These mechanisms exploit cognitive loopholes, tricking your brain into craving **just a little more**. And the longer you stay trapped in the loop, the more profitable your presence becomes.

## The Hidden Cost of "Free"

If a platform is free to use, **you're the product**. Every app, website, and social network that doesn't charge you upfront is making money in another way—by **selling access to your attention**. But it's not just your focus they're after—it's everything that comes with it.

Every click, search, and swipe feeds a larger system that tracks your behavior in microscopic detail. These data points—what you like, how long you watch, when you pause—are bundled and sold to advertisers hungry to target you with pinpoint accuracy. And it's not just surface-level data. Platforms track things you wouldn't expect—how fast you scroll, the words you hover over, even your emotional patterns. Over time, they build a profile that's not just about who you **are**, but who you're **becoming**.

The result? You're exposed to an ecosystem where every ad feels eerily relevant, every suggestion feels perfectly timed, and every impulse to engage feels almost **inevitable**. It's not magic—it's the byproduct of years of data collection, all aimed at making your attention a **predictable, sellable asset**.

What's unsettling is how little control you actually have over this process. Most data collection happens quietly, in the background, without you even realizing it. Your location history, your late-night searches, the products you almost bought but didn't—**it's all being tracked**. And once your attention becomes a measurable asset, your digital experience is no longer designed for you—it's designed for the advertisers who are paying to reach you.

## Your Time Is Priceless—But Not to Them

What's fascinating—and slightly terrifying—is how **cheaply** your time is sold. While platforms rake in billions of dollars, the average user's attention is worth mere **pennies per click**. Yet, those pennies add up. For companies that traffic in attention, even a fraction of a second is a revenue stream. And in a world where everyone is connected 24/7, those streams never stop flowing.

The real danger is what this does to your **sense of value**. When your focus is treated as a commodity, it's easy to lose sight of how precious it actually is. Your time isn't replaceable—it's the most **finite resource** you have. But when platforms design experiences that encourage mindless consumption, it's easy to trade hours of your day for nothing but fleeting entertainment and targeted ads.

And the scariest part? You probably don't even notice it happening. The algorithm's subtle nudges, the seamless transitions between content, the perfectly timed notifications—they're all designed to make your attention feel like it's **free to give**. But the truth is, every moment you spend locked in the loop is a moment you **can't get back**.

So how do you break free from a system designed to consume you? It starts with recognizing that **your attention is power**—and you don't have to give it away for free. Small shifts can disrupt the algorithm's hold on your focus. Try setting boundaries with your screen time, turning off non-essential notifications, or reclaiming your mornings before you reach for your phone.

And more importantly, start valuing your attention **the way they do**. Treat it like the precious, non-renewable resource it is. Be mindful of where your time goes—and who profits from it. Every second you reclaim is a step toward a life where your focus serves **you**, not the companies lining their pockets with it.

Because at the end of the day, your attention isn't just valuable to them—it's invaluable to **you**. And the moment you stop giving it away for free is the moment you start **taking back control**.

# 5

# The Endless Feed Illusion

IMAGINE SITTING DOWN WITH A bowl of your favourite snack. You plan to have just a few bites—but the bowl never empties. No matter how much you eat, there's always more. Sounds like a dream, right? Not quite. Psychologists call this the **bottomless bowl effect**, and it's a classic trick to make you consume more without realizing it. In the digital world, your endless scrolling isn't so different. Every time you swipe, there's another post, another video, another reason to stay. And like that never-ending bowl, it's not by accident—it's by **design**.

Infinite scrolling didn't just happen because technology advanced. It was carefully engineered to keep you **engaged longer**—and it works frighteningly well. Before endless feeds, you'd reach the end of a page, and that natural stopping point was a signal to **move on**. But platforms learned that if there's no bottom, there's no built-in cue to quit. So, they removed the endpoint entirely. Now, your social feeds, news platforms, and video apps are designed to feel **limitless**, blurring the line between casual browsing and compulsive consumption.

And it's not just keeping you entertained—it's keeping you **hooked**. Every time you think you're done, there's something new to discover. But here's the thing: you're not really choosing what you see. The illusion of endless content disguises a deeper reality—**you're being manipulated**. And the longer you scroll, the more this invisible design shapes not only your behaviour but also how you experience **time, choice, and even reality itself**.

## Why "Just One More" Feels So Hard to Resist

At the core of the endless feed illusion is a psychological trick called **variable reinforcement**—and it's the same mechanism behind slot machines. The idea is simple: when rewards are unpredictable, you become more **obsessed** with the next possible win. On social media, that win might be a funny meme, a heartwarming story, or a juicy piece of gossip. You don't know when it'll appear, so you keep scrolling. And because your brain is wired to chase unpredictable rewards, stopping feels almost **unnatural**.

This isn't an accident—it's an industry strategy. When you stay on a platform longer, you generate more data, see more ads, and become a more **valuable commodity**. That's why the most addictive platforms don't just offer content—they offer **infinite possibility**. Each scroll feels like opening a gift: maybe it'll be boring, or maybe it'll be mind-blowing. The uncertainty is what keeps you coming back.

And the scariest part? Your brain struggles to **recognize the trap**. With physical activities, there's a natural point where you stop—when you finish a book or a TV show, there's a clear end. But in a world where content never runs out, your brain's internal cues for "I'm done" get **short-circuited**. You lose track of time. You scroll longer than you intended. And suddenly, hours disappear into the black hole of your feed—leaving you drained but still wanting **more**.

## The Illusion of Choice

It feels like you're choosing what to watch, read, or engage with—but that's only part of the story. The truth is, algorithms decide what appears in your feed, and they're not designed to prioritize **what's good for you**. They're built to keep you on the platform. That means you're not actually in control—the algorithm is.

When you scroll, your options feel **endless**, but the reality is much narrower. You're shown content that fits your past behaviour and what the system predicts will hold your attention the longest. Ever notice how, after watching one video, you're served an avalanche of similar ones? That's not coincidence—it's **calculated**. The algorithm isn't giving you the full range of possibilities; it's giving you what's most **profitable**.

And while it feels like infinite choice, the truth is you're being subtly **guided**. The illusion of freedom masks the reality of manipulation. You think you're exploring at random—but your experience is being **curated** by forces you can't see. Every scroll, click, and pause teaches the system how to better **shape your desires**.

What's more unsettling is how easily this manipulation becomes **invisible**. When you're surrounded by content that feels tailor-made, it's easy to believe that you're just **following your interests**. But what happens when your feed limits what you encounter? You get trapped in an **echo chamber**—seeing the same ideas, the same opinions, and the same type of content on repeat. And while it feels like you're in charge, you're really following a **script** written by algorithms whose only goal is to hold your attention.

## How Infinite Feeds Distort Your Sense of Time

Ever opened your phone "just for a minute," only to realize an hour has vanished? That's no accident. Endless feeds blur the boundaries between **time well spent** and **time wasted**, tricking you into losing track of reality. And once you're inside the loop, time becomes slippery—stretched thin by an endless flow of content with no natural **stopping points**.

Part of the problem lies in how our brains process **closure**. Normally, we feel a sense of completion when we finish a task—whether it's reading a book, watching a movie, or completing a project. This sense of closure tells our brains, "You're done." But infinite feeds deny you that psychological release. Instead of a satisfying end, you face a **bottomless** well of new content, keeping your brain in a state of **anticipation**.

Without clear breaks, your internal clock gets disrupted. What felt like five minutes turns into fifty. This time distortion doesn't just affect your free time—it bleeds into your ability to focus, be present, and **engage with the real world**. The more you feed the scroll loop, the harder it becomes to **step outside** of it.

And here's the kicker: platforms know this. They know you're more likely to stick around when time feels **suspended**. So, they create environments where pauses and exits are harder to find—keeping you in a **perpetual now**, where there's always one more thing to see.

So, how do you escape a system built to make you **lose control**? It starts by seeing the illusion for what it is—a deliberate design choice that treats your attention as a **product**. Once you realize that your endless scrolling isn't about your choices but about **their profits**, the illusion starts to crack.

One powerful shift? **Create your own stopping points.** Since platforms won't offer you natural breaks, you have to set them yourself. Whether it's limiting your screen time, scheduling tech-free zones, or using external timers, these boundaries restore your sense of **control**.

And perhaps most importantly—**stay conscious**. Every time you open an app, remember: you're stepping into a space designed to hold you **captive**. By recognizing the psychological tricks at play, you reclaim the power to decide **when to stop**. Because in a world where your attention is currency, knowing when to walk away isn't just a skill—it's a form of **freedom**.

# 6

# Why Clicks Feel Like Cravings

YOU'RE MINDING YOUR BUSINESS, SCROLLING through your feed, and then it hits you. A headline so juicy, so outrageous, you can't resist. "You Won't Believe What Happened Next," "10 Secrets They Don't Want You to Know," "Is This the End of the World As We Know It?" You know it's clickbait. You know the answer probably won't be life-changing. And yet—**you click anyway**.

The pull isn't random. It's a psychological game, and you're not losing because you're weak. You're losing because the system is **rigged**. Every "irresistible" headline, viral video, or perfectly packaged post taps into ancient, hardwired impulses that your brain can't easily ignore. And the more you engage, the more these systems refine their ability to trigger your next click. But here's the twist—it's not just about what you see. It's about how the internet learned to **hack your cravings** and turn them into profit.

At the core of clickbait is one simple principle: **curiosity gaps**. It's the space between what you know and what you *want* to know. And your brain? It hates the gap. When there's missing information—especially when it feels like a secret—you're wired to **fill the void**. It's the same itch that makes you lean in when someone says, "I probably shouldn't tell you this…"

Researchers call this the **Zeigarnik effect**—the tendency to fixate on unfinished tasks or unanswered questions. When a headline dangles something mysterious or incomplete, your brain perceives it as **unfinished business**. And once you're hooked, you'll click, swipe, and scroll until that tension is resolved. Platforms know this, and they weaponize it. Every vague headline or dramatic thumbnail is crafted to **poke at that gap**—and once they have your attention, they're not letting go.

What's worse? The emotional charge of clickbait makes the craving stronger. Your brain lights up for **emotional extremes**—whether it's shock, outrage, or awe. And clickbait headlines are designed to deliver precisely that. It's not about delivering useful information—it's about keeping you in a heightened state where **curiosity overrides common sense**.

And it works. Studies show that emotionally charged content spreads faster and further than neutral content. Rage-inducing headlines get **17% more clicks**, while sensationalism boosts engagement across every platform. This isn't just an accident—it's a business model.

## Why Your Brain Loves the Drama

You might think you're drawn to clickbait because you're curious—but the truth is deeper. The human brain evolved in environments where **threat detection** was essential to survival. Being attuned to dramatic or unexpected events helped our ancestors avoid danger, secure resources, and stay alive. In today's digital age, that instinct still exists—but instead of scanning the savannah for predators, we're scrolling through **feeds of manufactured drama**.

This craving for the sensational is amplified by how your brain processes **reward**. Every time you click on a juicy headline, your brain releases a hit of **dopamine**—the neurotransmitter responsible for pleasure and motivation. But here's the catch: it's not the *satisfaction* of getting answers that hooks you—it's the

**anticipation**. That surge of dopamine spikes **before** you click, creating a craving for the reward that keeps you coming back for more.

And, just like with other addictive behaviours, your brain starts to **re-wire** itself. The more you engage with clickbait, the more your brain associates that behaviour with **instant gratification**. Over time, it becomes harder to resist—even when you know it's a trap.

Ever wonder why you can't stop watching outrage-fueled debates or scanning celebrity gossip? That's not just personal weakness—it's **neuroscience in action**. Platforms don't just know this—they're **banking on it**.

## The Science of Viral Content

Behind every viral headline and trending video is a carefully calculated system. It's not just about creating content—it's about creating content that your brain finds **irresistible**. And while it might feel random, the science behind viral content is **deeply deliberate**.

For starters, viral content typically hits on at least **one** of these psychological triggers:

- **Emotion** – The stronger the feeling (joy, anger, fear), the more likely you are to click and share.
- **Surprise** – Unexpected twists stimulate your brain's novelty-seeking circuits.
- **Identity** – Content that aligns with your beliefs or worldview feels **personal**—and share-worthy.
- **Fear of Missing Out (FOMO)** – If everyone else is talking about it, your brain doesn't want to be left behind.

Platforms use sophisticated AI to test and optimize content in

**real-time**—tracking which headlines get the most clicks, which emotions drive the strongest responses, and which stories make people stick around. The result? A **feedback loop** where the most addictive content gets pushed to the top—while everything else fades into the background.

And you? You're caught in a cycle where your clicks teach the algorithm **how to bait you better**.

## Breaking the Clickbait Cycle

Here's the hard truth: you're not going to out-willpower a system designed to outsmart you. The only way to regain control is to **disrupt the craving loop**.

Start by recognizing the emotional **hooks**. Next time you feel the itch to click on something sensational, pause and ask:

*What emotion is this triggering?*

*Do I actually care about the content—or just the curiosity gap?*

By becoming aware of these tactics, you can start to **short-circuit** their hold on you. You're not powerless—but you have to become **conscious**.

Another game-changer? **Limit your exposure to engineered triggers.** Unfollow sensational accounts. Use browser extensions to block clickbait-heavy sites. And when you catch yourself spiraling into curiosity traps, pull yourself out by **reclaiming your focus**.

And finally—remember **why** these tricks exist in the first place. Your attention isn't just being captured—it's being **monetized**. Every click is a data point. Every share feeds the system. The less you engage with engineered drama, the less power these algorithms have over your behaviour.

At the end of the day, clickbait works because it exploits a **deeply human craving** for answers and emotional highs. But once you start to see the game for what it is, you can choose to play by **your own rules**. Your brain might love the bait—but you don't have to bite.

# 7

# Fast Content, Slow Brain

IN A WORLD WHERE EVERYTHING moves at hyper-speed, your brain is running a marathon it never signed up for. You open TikTok "just for five minutes," and suddenly it's two hours later, your thumb is sore, and your brain feels like it's been through a blender. The rapid-fire nature of short-form content isn't just harmless entertainment—it's **changing how you think, focus, and even feel**. And the scariest part? It's doing it without you even noticing.

When you're bombarded with 15-second clips, your brain adapts to a rhythm where **everything needs to be fast, flashy, and instantly gratifying**. But while the content is speeding up, your cognitive ability to process and retain information? **It's slowing down**. It's not just about what you watch—it's about how this constant stream of fast content is rewiring the very foundation of how you engage with the world. And the long-term consequences? They're way more serious than just losing a few hours in a TikTok black hole.

It's not in your imagination—your attention span is shrinking. Research suggests that over the past two decades, the average human attention span has **dropped from 12 seconds to just 8 seconds**—that's less than a goldfish. And short-form platforms like TikTok, Instagram Reels, and YouTube Shorts? They're accelerating that decline.

The reason lies in how **your brain processes information**. Every time you consume fast, bite-sized content, your brain gets better at handling **quick bursts of stimulation** but worse at managing **sustained focus**. Think of it like training a muscle. If all you ever do are quick sprints, you'll struggle to run a marathon. And when you're scrolling through a feed where every video is shorter, snappier, and more stimulating than the last, your brain becomes hooked on **instant gratification**—and struggles with anything requiring **patience or deep thought**.

And the effects are more than just mental fatigue. Studies show that regular consumption of fast content is linked to **higher levels of anxiety, reduced working memory, and increased impulsivity**. It's not just making you more distracted—it's making it harder to think critically, process complex ideas, and stay present in your daily life.

But here's the kicker: these platforms **know** what they're doing. The algorithms are designed to reward content that's **fast, engaging, and easy to consume**—not content that requires thought, reflection, or depth. And once your brain adjusts to this quick-hit cycle, it starts to crave **more of the same**. The result? You get stuck in a loop where slower, deeper forms of engagement—like reading a book or having a long conversation—feel **boring** in comparison.

## Information Overload in Real-Time

When you scroll through rapid-fire videos, your brain isn't just passively absorbing information—it's working **overtime**. Each new clip triggers your brain's **dopamine system**, releasing tiny hits of pleasure with every swipe. But unlike natural rewards (like eating a great meal or laughing with a friend), digital dopamine is **cheap and easy**—and your brain knows it.

The constant flood of stimuli forces your brain to make **micro-decisions** at lightning speed: Do I watch this? Swipe past it? Like it? Share it? And while this might seem harmless, over time, it **exhausts your cognitive resources**. Your brain becomes less efficient at processing new information, and the ability to focus on **a single, uninterrupted task** takes a serious hit.

And it's not just about focus—it's about how your brain categorizes and stores information. Short-form content **fragments your thinking**, making it harder to connect ideas, remember important details, or engage in deep reflection. Instead of processing knowledge in a cohesive narrative, your brain becomes flooded with **disjointed snippets**—random facts, half-formed ideas, and fleeting impressions.

The result? You start living in a state of **perpetual mental chaos**—where everything feels urgent, nothing feels meaningful, and your ability to process life in **real time** gets slower by the day.

## Why Deep Thinking Feels Impossible

Ever notice how reading a book or focusing on a long article feels harder than it used to? That's not just an attention issue— it's a **neuroplasticity** issue. Your brain is constantly reshaping itself based on how you use it. The more you train your mind for **short bursts of attention**, the harder it becomes to engage in **slow, reflective thinking**.

And it's not just affecting how you consume content—it's changing how you engage with the **real world**. Conversations feel harder to follow. Boredom feels unbearable. Waiting in line without pulling out your phone? Unthinkable. Your brain is constantly seeking the **next hit**, making quiet moments feel uncomfortable—even though they're essential for **mental clarity and emotional regulation**.

In a culture obsessed with speed, **slowing down** feels counterintuitive. But without space for **deep thought**, your ability to make sound decisions, engage creatively, and maintain emotional resilience gets weaker. The brain you bring to TikTok isn't the brain you need to **thrive in real life**—and the longer you stay hooked on fast content, the harder it becomes to switch gears.

## The Case for Slow Consumption

Here's the truth: **you don't have to quit** short-form content to protect your brain—but you do need to break the fast-content cycle. And it starts by retraining your mind to slow down and engage more deliberately.

One of the most powerful interventions? Digital fasting—intentional breaks from high-speed content that give your brain a chance to reset. Research shows that even short periods of digital detoxing can improve focus, memory, and overall cognitive function. By limiting your exposure to rapid-fire media, you give your brain space to rebuild the neural pathways needed for deeper thought.

Another game-changer? Slow media consumption. Prioritize content that demands attention and patience—whether it's long-form writing, podcasts with depth, or even in-person conversations. When you engage with slower, more reflective forms of media, you strengthen the parts of your brain responsible for critical thinking and emotional regulation.

And finally—practice boredom. Let your mind wander without distraction. Give yourself permission to sit in silence. These moments aren't wasted time—they're essential for helping your brain integrate information and restore mental balance.

The TikTok Effect is real—but it's not irreversible. By choosing to engage more consciously, you can reclaim your ability to think deeply, focus fully, and live in the present moment. Your brain might love fast content—but your mind deserves something better.

# 8

# Why Doomscrolling Feels So Good (Until It Doesn't)

IT'S 11:47 P.M., AND YOU tell yourself you'll check the news "just for a second." Fast-forward an hour, and you're still glued to your phone, spiraling through a black hole of bad headlines. Political chaos, climate disasters, economic uncertainty—each story worse than the last, and yet, you **can't stop scrolling**. Your eyes burn, your heart races, but you keep going. It's not that you enjoy feeling stressed—it's that your brain, against all logic, **wants more**.

Doomscrolling isn't just a bad habit—it's **a biological trap**. Your brain is wired to pay attention to potential threats, and the internet is a never-ending buffet of worst-case scenarios. Each headline feels urgent, like you might miss something vital if you stop. And while you scroll in search of clarity or reassurance, what you actually get is a steady drip of **anxiety, helplessness, and emotional fatigue**. So, why does it feel so good in the moment— and so awful afterward? The answer lies deep in your brain's obsession with **negative information** and the illusion of control that doomscrolling promises but never delivers.

## Your Brain Is Addicted to Bad News

Humans have a built-in negativity bias—a psychological quirk that makes us **pay more attention to threats than positive information**. Back when life involved outrunning predators, this bias was a survival advantage. Fast-forward to today, and that same instinct means your brain treats **bad news like life-or-death information**, even when it's just another headline.

When you scroll through negative content, your brain floods with **stress hormones** like cortisol and adrenaline—chemicals designed to keep you alert and ready for action. But here's the twist: that stress also triggers your **dopamine system**, the same reward pathway activated by sugar, drugs, and social media likes. So, each time you stumble on a terrifying headline, your brain rewards you with a hit of dopamine, reinforcing the behavior and making you **want to keep scrolling**.

And the internet? It knows this. Algorithms prioritize **sensational, fear-inducing content** because it keeps you engaged longer. The scarier and more urgent the story, the more likely you are to click, share, and—most importantly—**stay hooked**. You think you're staying informed, but what you're really doing is **feeding an addiction loop** that thrives on your anxiety.

## Why You Keep Scrolling

Doomscrolling feels productive. It tricks your brain into thinking that if you just **consume enough information**, you'll regain some sense of control over the chaos. This is especially true during times of crisis—whether it's a global pandemic, a political upheaval, or a personal emergency. Your brain craves **certainty**, and the internet promises a never-ending stream of updates that seem to offer answers.

But here's the catch: **the more you scroll, the less in control you actually feel**. Studies show that consuming excessive negative news increases feelings of **helplessness, anxiety, and depression**.

Instead of making you feel informed, it overwhelms your brain with problems you can't solve, reinforcing a sense that the world is spiraling while you're stuck, powerless to stop it.

Worse still, doomscrolling disrupts your brain's ability to **distinguish between actual threats and hypothetical ones**. Your nervous system doesn't know the difference between reading about a disaster and living through one—so every terrifying headline activates your **fight-or-flight** response. The result? Chronic stress that lingers long after you've put your phone down.

## The Emotional Toll of Constant Digital Dread

The effects of doomscrolling don't end when you stop scrolling. Over time, constant exposure to bad news reshapes your emotional landscape, leaving you more anxious, cynical, and exhausted. Research shows that prolonged consumption of distressing content can lead to **hyper-vigilance**—a state where your brain is constantly on high alert, scanning for danger even in safe environments.

This hyper-vigilance can bleed into everyday life. You might find yourself checking your phone compulsively, struggling to relax, or feeling a low-level sense of dread even when nothing is wrong. Your brain, conditioned to expect bad news, starts to interpret **neutral situations as threatening**, making it harder to trust good things when they happen.

And the emotional fallout doesn't stop there. Doomscrolling can disrupt your **sleep cycle**, leaving you wired and restless long after bedtime. It can damage your ability to **focus**, as your brain becomes addicted to the constant novelty of new information. And perhaps most concerning—it can numb your emotional responses. When you're exposed to crisis after crisis, your brain eventually **desensitizes** itself as a defense mechanism, making it harder to feel empathy, joy, or even concern.

In other words, the longer you stay trapped in the doomscrolling cycle, the harder it becomes to **feel anything fully**—good or bad.

## How to Reclaim Your Mind

Here's the truth: **you can't out-scroll anxiety**. No amount of information will give you the sense of control you're craving. The only way to break free from the doomscrolling trap is to **interrupt the cycle**—to stop feeding your brain a diet of endless dread and start engaging with information in a way that **protects your mental and emotional health**.

One of the most powerful tools? **Digital boundaries.** Set limits on how and when you consume news—whether it's giving yourself a "scroll curfew" or choosing specific, reliable sources rather than falling into the algorithm's rabbit hole. When you're intentional about your media intake, you create **mental space** for rest, reflection, and emotional recovery.

It also helps to **retrain your brain** by balancing your information diet. For every negative story you consume, seek out **positive or solution-focused content**—research shows this can reduce feelings of helplessness and increase optimism. Your brain needs evidence that **good things are still happening**, even when the world feels like it's on fire.

And when the urge to scroll hits, **pause** and check in with yourself: What am I really looking for? Reassurance? Distraction? Control? Often, naming the emotion behind the behavior can weaken its grip. Instead of mindlessly consuming more bad news, engage in activities that ground you—whether it's a walk outside, a conversation with someone you love, or simply **turning your phone off** and giving your brain room to breathe.

Doomscrolling feels good—until it doesn't. But you're not powerless against the pull. With a little intention and a lot of self-compassion, you can break free from the digital dread trap and reclaim your **peace of mind**.

PART 2

# The Psychological Games
# You Didn't Sign Up For

# 9

# Why You're Always Mad Online

LOG ON, AND THERE IT is—a fresh controversy, a viral fight, and a thousand hot takes demanding your attention. Within minutes, you're sucked in. Heart pounding, fingers flying, you're drafting the perfect response or scrolling through an endless sea of people arguing in the comments. You feel angry, righteous, and weirdly energized. And even though it drains you, you can't seem to look away. It's not just you—the internet is designed to make you mad, and it's not an accident.

At the heart of this phenomenon lies the outrage machine—a system where platforms profit from your anger because it's one of the most powerful drivers of engagement. When you're mad, you click more, comment more, and stay online longer. And every second you spend caught in the chaos is another opportunity for tech companies to collect data and sell ads. It's not about fostering real conversation—it's about keeping you hooked on conflict as entertainment. But here's the kicker: while the machine feeds off your anger, it's quietly reshaping your brain, your relationships, and the way you see the world.

Anger spreads faster than joy.

Emotionally, anger is like caffeine for the brain—fast, stimulating, and hard to ignore. It activates your amygdala, the part of the brain responsible for processing threats, making you hyper-focused and ready to react. Unlike joy or curiosity, which foster calm, anger triggers your fight response, pushing you to engage in an attempt to "correct" the perceived wrong.

And because our brains are wired to prioritize threats over neutral or positive information, anger-based content spreads like wildfire. Studies show that outrage posts—those dripping with moral indignation—are shared and commented on at a far higher rate than anything else. Algorithms, trained to prioritize engagement, push this content to the top of your feed because it keeps you on the platform longer. Every time you react, you reinforce the system, teaching it that outrage is what you want— even if it's quietly exhausting you.

The more you consume outrage content, the easier it becomes for your brain to expect and seek it out. It's called emotional priming—once your brain is tuned to anger, you start perceiving neutral or ambiguous situations as hostile. So that petty tweet or offhand comment? It hits you harder. And the longer you stay in the cycle, the more emotionally reactive you become, even offline.

## How Platforms Reward and Amplify Outrage

Social media isn't a neutral space—it's a carefully engineered environment designed to manipulate your emotions. The algorithm doesn't care whether you're happy, sad, or furious— it only cares about engagement metrics. And nothing drives engagement quite like rage.

Take the classic structure of viral outrage: an inflammatory post, a wave of angry responses, and a counter-wave of people calling out the original poster. This cycle is predictable, and platforms know it. Features like quote tweets, reaction buttons, and trending hashtags are built to escalate conflict, turning every disagreement into a public spectacle. You're not just a user—you're an unpaid actor in a digital drama, one where tech companies get richer every time you engage.

But the real kicker? Outrage isn't just profitable—it's contagious. Research shows that exposure to angry content primes you to produce angry content yourself. So when you see a post that makes your blood boil, your brain shifts into retaliation mode, making you more likely to post something sharp, snarky, or aggressive. This isn't just a psychological quirk—it's a system working as intended, keeping the outrage machine well-oiled and unstoppable.

## The Psychological Toll of Constant Conflict

Here's what the outrage machine doesn't tell you: being mad all the time is exhausting. Chronic exposure to anger spikes your cortisol levels—the hormone responsible for stress—leaving you wired, tense, and emotionally depleted. Over time, this constant state of reactivity wears down your mental resilience, increasing your risk for anxiety, depression, and burnout.

And the toll isn't just internal—it also affects your relationships. When your brain is primed for conflict, you become quicker to judge, slower to empathize, and more likely to interpret others' words or actions as malicious. Conversations feel heavier, misunderstandings escalate faster, and the sense of connection frays. The more time you spend consuming and participating in outrage, the harder it becomes to access nuance, making everything feel black-and-white—even when reality is far more complex.

Worse still, the outrage cycle traps you in a dopamine loop. That rush you feel when you fire off a heated reply? That's your brain rewarding you for "defending" yourself. But like any high, the relief is temporary—and soon, you're back scrolling for the next thing to get mad about, feeding a cycle that drains your energy while giving nothing in return.

## Breaking the Outrage Consumption Loop

So, how do you reclaim your peace when the internet is designed to keep you angry? It starts with disrupting the pattern—recognizing when you're being baited and stepping off the outrage treadmill before it pulls you in.

One of the most effective tools is emotional distance. When you encounter something inflammatory, pause before reacting. Ask yourself: Is this worth my energy? Often, outrage posts are designed to provoke, not inform—and refusing to engage deprives the algorithm of the fuel it needs to keep spreading the fire.

Another strategy? Curate your digital environment. Mute, unfollow, or block sources that consistently amplify conflict without offering solutions. Prioritize content that informs without inflaming—spaces where real dialogue happens, not just performative outrage. Your feed is your mental diet, and the cleaner it is, the better your emotional health will be.

Finally, practice empathy over immediacy. The internet encourages snap judgments and quick reactions, but real understanding takes time. When faced with a controversial topic, seek out multiple perspectives instead of relying on algorithm-driven soundbites. Not everything deserves your anger—and when you protect your peace, you regain the mental clarity to focus on the things that actually matter.

The outrage machine wants your attention—but you don't have to give it. When you break free from the cycle, you reclaim not just your time, but your emotional freedom—and that's a power no algorithm can take away.

# 10

## Fear Sells

IF YOU'VE EVER FOUND YOURSELF glued to your screen during a breaking news event—refreshing updates, diving into endless threads, feeling your heart rate climb—you've felt the power of fear-based content in action. It's a familiar loop: an alarming headline grabs your attention, your anxiety spikes, and suddenly, you're deep in a vortex of worst-case scenarios. Even when you know it's stressing you out, stepping away feels impossible. And that's not an accident. Fear isn't just a natural human response—it's a business model in the digital age.

In a world where attention equals profit, fear is a goldmine. It's potent, sticky, and incredibly effective at keeping you engaged. Platforms thrive on emotional intensity, and nothing holds your focus like a looming crisis. From sensationalist headlines to dramatic push notifications, the digital ecosystem is built to hijack your survival instincts, turning every potential threat into a must-click emergency. But while fear-based content drives record engagement, it also wreaks havoc on your mental state, leaving you trapped in a cycle of panic, paranoia, and powerlessness.

To understand why fear sells so well, you have to start with evolution. Your brain is wired to prioritize threat detection—a survival mechanism known as negativity bias. Back when our ancestors roamed the wild, missing a potential danger (like a predator) could mean death, so our brains evolved to pay extra attention to negative stimuli. Fast forward to today, and that same mechanism kicks in every time you see a headline screaming about global disasters, economic collapse, or an impending apocalypse.

The media knows this—and exploits it. Fear activates your amygdala, the brain's emotional alarm system, flooding your system with adrenaline and hijacking your focus. You're hardwired to keep scanning for more information to assess the threat, which means you're more likely to click, scroll, and stay glued to crisis coverage for hours. And the scarier the content, the harder it is to resist. This is why phrases like "breaking news," "crisis," and "urgent warning" dominate your feed—they're engineered to trip your brain's fear circuits and keep you locked in.

But it's not just about grabbing your attention—it's about holding it. Platforms use intermittent reinforcement—the same psychological principle behind slot machines—to keep you engaged. Every refresh brings the possibility of new, anxiety-inducing information, creating a feedback loop where your brain becomes addicted to checking for the latest updates. The more you scroll, the more you teach your brain that constant vigilance is necessary for survival—even when the actual threat is far removed from your daily reality.

## The Science of Panic Scrolling During Crises

When a crisis hits—whether it's a global pandemic or a political upheaval—the urge to panic-scroll becomes almost irresistible. You might tell yourself that you're staying informed, but what's really happening is an overload of threat signals flooding your brain. This triggers your sympathetic nervous system, the body's fight-or-flight response, leaving you in a heightened state of stress and hypervigilance.

Research shows that consuming high volumes of distressing media during a crisis increases symptoms of anxiety, depression, and PTSD—even for people not directly affected by the event. Your brain can't always distinguish between virtual danger and real-life threat, which means that absorbing catastrophic content can feel as overwhelming as living through it. And the longer you engage, the harder it becomes to switch off.

What's more? Crisis content often plays on anticipatory fear— the dread of something bad that hasn't happened yet. This is why you'll see headlines laced with speculative phrases like "could lead to," "potential disaster," and "experts warn." These vague but alarming predictions create a sense of perpetual uncertainty, pushing your brain to keep seeking more information in a desperate attempt to regain a sense of control. But instead of clarity, you end up drowning in a sea of worst-case scenarios— exhausted, but unable to stop.

## Why Fear-Based Algorithms Thrive in Uncertain Times

Fear isn't just psychologically potent—it's profitable. During times of uncertainty, engagement spikes across the board. People spend more time online, click more headlines, and dive deeper into social feeds looking for reassurance. Platforms and news outlets know this, and their algorithms adapt accordingly. Content that triggers strong emotions—especially fear—gets boosted to the top because it drives the most user interaction.

This means that in a crisis, your feed becomes a fear amplifier. Algorithms prioritize emotionally charged posts—the ones that get people arguing, sharing, and obsessing. And the scarier the story, the further it spreads. What you see isn't an objective reflection of reality—it's a curated fearscape designed to keep you hooked.

But here's the dark side: prolonged exposure to fear-driven content can warp your perception of the world. It heightens your risk sensitivity, making everyday situations feel more dangerous than they are. Over time, you may begin to view the world through a lens of chronic threat, where even small uncertainties feel like impending disasters. And while the algorithm profits from your prolonged attention, you're left feeling helpless and emotionally drained.

Escaping the fear trap doesn't mean tuning out the world—but it does mean reclaiming control over how and when you engage with crisis content. It's about protecting your mental bandwidth without falling prey to manipulative fear tactics.

First, set boundaries around your information diet. Limit your exposure to panic-driven platforms and choose sources known for measured, factual reporting over sensationalism. Curate your feed intentionally—unfollow accounts that traffic in anxiety and prioritize content that provides context instead of chaos.

Second, schedule check-ins instead of doomscrolling. Designate specific times to catch up on news rather than letting crisis content ambush you throughout the day. This not only reduces emotional fatigue but also helps you stay grounded in reality instead of drowning in hypothetical catastrophes.

Another powerful tool? Mindful consumption. When you feel the urge to dive into panic-scrolling, pause and ask yourself: Is this information useful, or is it just making me anxious? Recognize when the algorithm is feeding your fears and disrupt the cycle by stepping away.

And finally, anchor yourself in reality. Fear-based content thrives on vagueness and speculation—but your brain craves certainty. When a headline triggers anxiety, seek real data and trusted experts rather than social media rumors. The more you ground yourself in facts over fear, the harder it becomes for manipulative algorithms to control your emotional state.

In a world where fear sells, staying calm is an act of rebellion. By reclaiming your focus and refusing to feed the fear machine, you take back your time, your peace of mind, and—most importantly—your power.

# 11

# How Constant Alerts Keep You on Edge

PICTURE THIS: YOU'RE FINALLY SETTLING into a quiet moment, your brain just starting to unwind—when your phone buzzes. A message. Another buzz. An email. Before you know it, you're back in the loop, bouncing between apps, checking notifications you swear you'll "just glance at," and wondering why you constantly feel on edge. It's not just you—your nervous system is under siege. Every ping, buzz, and alert is more than a minor disruption. It's a carefully crafted mechanism designed to pull you back in, flood your brain with stimulation, and keep you hooked on the cycle of anxiety.

Modern technology didn't just give us instant access to information—it created a world where constant availability is expected. And while those tiny red dots may seem harmless, the truth is that every notification is a psychological trigger, priming your brain to stay on high alert. From social media mentions to urgent-sounding emails, the endless stream of digital prompts isn't just exhausting—it's fundamentally rewiring how you experience stress.

Your brain is an ancient machine navigating a modern maze. At its core, it's designed to detect and respond to threats—a survival instinct called the fight-or-flight response. While your ancestors faced predators in the wild, your brain now reacts to a different kind of intruder: your phone. Every notification, no matter how trivial, activates your sympathetic nervous system— the part of your brain responsible for that heart-pounding, hyper-alert feeling.

Research shows that even a silent notification triggers a physiological response. Your heart rate increases, your cortisol levels spike, and your body prepares for action. This is why a simple email alert can feel as urgent as a real-life emergency. Over time, these micro-stressors accumulate, creating a state of chronic low-grade anxiety. You may not even realize it, but your body stays in a constant state of readiness, always anticipating the next interruption.

And it doesn't stop there. The unpredictability of notifications makes them even more addictive. This is called variable reinforcement—the same principle that drives gambling addiction. You never know when the next notification will be rewarding (a fun message) or stressful (an urgent work email), so your brain learns to stay alert just in case. This unpredictability heightens your stress response and keeps you checking, even when you don't want to.

## The Psychology of "Always-On" Culture

Beyond the physical stress, there's a deeper psychological toll: the pressure of being constantly available. In a world where notifications blur the line between work and personal life, switching off feels like a luxury most people can't afford. The expectation to respond instantly—whether to a boss's email or a friend's text—creates a sense of perpetual urgency, even when nothing is actually urgent.

Psychologists call this phenomenon "telepressure"—the feeling that you must respond to digital communications immediately. This pressure erodes your ability to relax because your brain never gets the signal that it's safe to fully disengage. Instead of winding down, you stay mentally tethered to your devices, always bracing for the next demand on your attention. And the more you engage, the harder it is to resist.

This always-on culture also blurs the boundary between public and private life. Notifications drag external demands into your most intimate moments—dinner with friends, bedtime rituals, even moments of self-reflection. Your brain loses the ability to differentiate between personal space and public urgency, leading to cognitive overload—the mental exhaustion that comes from processing too much information, too fast.

And it's not just about the big alerts—micro-interruptions matter, too. Studies show that even a quick glance at a notification can disrupt your focus for up to 25 minutes. This means that every buzz fractures your attention, leaving you mentally scattered and emotionally drained. And the irony? Most notifications aren't even urgent—but your brain treats them all as if they are.

## How to Manage Alert Fatigue and Reclaim Mental Space

If you feel like your brain is constantly being hijacked by notifications, you're not imagining it. Alert fatigue is a very real thing, and it's a form of cognitive exhaustion caused by constant interruptions. Over time, this mental overload reduces your ability to focus deeply, process information, and regulate your emotions.

One of the first steps to breaking free from the anxiety algorithm is to take back control of your notifications—because right now, they're controlling you. This doesn't mean going full digital detox (unless that's your vibe). It's about being intentional with what gets access to your attention.

Start by prioritizing your alerts. Not everything deserves a buzz. Identify the notifications that are actually important (like genuine emergencies) and silence the rest. Disable non-essential alerts—think social media likes, marketing emails, and random app updates. You don't need to know every time someone uploads a story or your favorite shopping app drops a sale.

Next, try batching your notifications. Instead of letting alerts trickle in all day, set specific times to check them. This technique, known as notification batching, helps reduce the frequency of interruptions, giving your brain the downtime it craves. Imagine the difference between being poked constantly and getting all your updates in one go—it's the mental equivalent of peace and quiet.

And here's the game-changer: Do Not Disturb Mode is your best friend. Use it liberally—especially during key focus periods, relaxation time, or before bed. Studies show that people who limit digital interruptions experience lower stress levels and improved cognitive functioning. Give your brain the break it deserves.

## Why Unplugging Improves Emotional Regulation

Constant alerts don't just disrupt your focus—they mess with your emotions, too. Every time your brain switches from calm to alert mode, it disrupts your ability to process feelings in a balanced way. This is why spending too much time reacting to notifications can leave you feeling anxious, irritable, and overwhelmed—even when there's no external reason for it.

Unplugging—whether it's for an hour, an afternoon, or a whole weekend—gives your brain a chance to reset. When you reduce digital noise, your nervous system gets to exit the fight-or-flight cycle and return to a state of rest and digest. This not only improves your emotional stability but also strengthens your focus, creativity, and overall mental clarity.

But unplugging is about more than just turning off your phone—it's about reclaiming your attention as a form of power. Every time you choose to disengage from the noise, you're telling the world: my peace isn't for sale. In a culture that profits from your distraction, choosing stillness is a radical act.

So, the next time your phone lights up with yet another alert, ask yourself: Is this worth my peace of mind? Because the truth is, your attention is yours to give—or to take back.

# 12

# When Everyone Else's Life Looks Better

IT STARTS WITH AN INNOCENT scroll—someone's vacation in Bali, another's engagement ring, a perfect Sunday brunch with friends. Before you know it, you're knee-deep in curated perfection, wondering why your own life suddenly feels a little less exciting. Welcome to comparison culture, where everyone else's life seems shinier, happier, and far more effortless—at least through the lens of social media.

Humans have always compared themselves to others—it's part of how we learn, measure our progress, and find our place in the world. But social media has taken this age-old instinct and supercharged it, serving up a never-ending stream of filtered realities that blur the line between inspiration and inadequacy. The problem isn't just that we compare—it's that we're comparing our raw, unedited lives to the highlight reels of everyone else. And in a world where perfection sells, the reality behind the screen often gets lost.

Your brain is wired to compare—it's a feature, not a bug. Psychologists call it social comparison theory, the idea that we evaluate our own worth by measuring ourselves against others. In prehistoric times, these comparisons helped us survive—knowing where you stood in the tribe could mean the difference between thriving and being left behind. But today, that instinct has evolved into something far more insidious, fueled by constant digital exposure.

The brain doesn't distinguish between what's relevant and what's not—it just compares. Whether it's a stranger's vacation photos or your best friend's job promotion, your mind automatically processes this information as a benchmark. And because your brain is hardwired to focus on what's missing, these comparisons often leave you feeling like you're falling short—no matter how well you're actually doing.

What makes social media comparisons especially potent is the sheer volume. In the past, you might have compared yourself to your immediate social circle. Now, you're exposed to thousands of people's curated lives every single day. And the result? A constant sense of not measuring up, even when you know—deep down—that the images you're consuming are only half the truth.

## The Illusion of Perfection in Curated Content

Let's be real—no one's life is as flawless as it looks online. Behind every dreamy vacation photo is a delayed flight or a missed connection. That glowing selfie? Probably the result of good lighting, 37 takes, and a little post-editing magic. But here's the catch: your brain doesn't always recognize the edits. It sees the polished version and assumes that's reality—and the more you consume, the easier it is to believe that everyone else has it figured out except you.

Social media thrives on curation—the careful selection of moments that present a perfectly packaged version of life. And while there's nothing inherently wrong with sharing highlights, the constant exposure to curated content creates a perception gap. You see someone's best day while living your average one, and the contrast makes your reality feel... less.

This illusion of perfection is especially dangerous because it magnifies insecurities you didn't even know you had. Suddenly, your perfectly fine apartment feels too small compared to someone's Pinterest-worthy loft. Your relationship—solid and loving—feels less romantic because it doesn't come with grand gestures for the 'gram. It's not that your life is lacking—it's that you're measuring it against an impossible standard.

And the platforms know this. The more you compare, the more you scroll—hoping to close the gap between your reality and the perfection you're chasing. The algorithm profits from your insecurity, feeding you endless images of lives that seem just out of reach, while leaving you to wonder why your own feels like it's falling behind.

## How Comparison Fuels Dissatisfaction and Self-Doubt

It's not just your mood that takes a hit—comparison culture directly impacts your mental health. Studies consistently show that heavy social media use correlates with increased anxiety, depression, and low self-esteem, especially when you're using it to compare your life to others.

One of the most damaging effects of comparison is the erosion of self-worth. Every time you measure yourself against someone else's success, beauty, or lifestyle, you reinforce the belief that you're not enough. And because social media only shows the best bits, you're left comparing your struggles to everyone else's highlights—a game you'll always lose.

Even when you know it's not real, the emotional impact lingers. Seeing a peer's rapid career climb can trigger feelings of failure, even if you're making progress on your own terms. Watching someone document their seemingly perfect relationship might make you question your own, despite its depth and authenticity. The more you compare, the harder it becomes to appreciate what you already have—because someone, somewhere, always seems to have more.

And here's the sneaky part: comparison doesn't stop once you "catch up." If you finally get the dream job, the perfect body, or the ideal vacation, social media will always show you someone doing it bigger, better, or sooner. The finish line keeps moving, ensuring that satisfaction is always just out of reach.

## Ways to Disrupt the Social Media Comparison Trap

The good news? You don't have to play the comparison game—at least, not on the internet's terms. Reclaiming your peace starts with recognizing when you're being pulled into the trap and disrupting the cycle before it spirals.

First, curate your feed with intention. Unfollow or mute accounts that trigger feelings of inadequacy. It doesn't mean you're bitter—it means you're protecting your mental health. Instead, surround yourself with content that reflects realness and diversity—the messy, beautiful, unfiltered parts of life.

Next, remind yourself of the behind-the-scenes reality. No one's life is perfect—even if their grid is. When you catch yourself feeling envious, pause and ask: What's the full story I'm not seeing? That glossy vacation photo doesn't show the arguments, the budget stress, or the 4 AM airport scramble. Context matters, and reminding yourself of the unseen truths takes the power out of comparison.

And perhaps most importantly, ground yourself in gratitude. Comparison thrives on scarcity—on the belief that there's not enough joy, success, or love to go around. But the truth is, your life is already full of enough, if you're willing to see it. Regularly reflecting on what you cherish shifts your focus from what's missing to what's present, creating a sense of abundance that no Instagram feed can take away.

Finally, give yourself permission to step back. Social media is a tool—not a mirror. You don't have to be always online to be relevant, lovable, or enough. The most meaningful parts of life? They're happening beyond the scroll, in the quiet, unfiltered moments that no algorithm can capture. And that's where your real value lies.

# 13

# Why Online Fights Feel
# So Personal

YOU TELL YOURSELF YOU'RE JUST "checking notifications," but somehow, you end up neck-deep in a heated comment thread. Your heart's racing, fingers flying, and suddenly—you're in a full-blown digital showdown with a stranger who, let's be honest, probably wouldn't say half of this to your face. It's the internet's version of a bar fight—except no one's throwing punches, and everyone's ego is on the line. But why does online conflict hit so differently? And why is it so hard to log off when things get messy?

At its core, the internet has turned disagreements into public performances. Arguments that once happened behind closed doors now unfold in front of an audience—an audience that likes, shares, and sometimes eggs things on. The stakes feel higher because, in a digital space, you're not just defending your opinion—you're defending your identity. Every comment feels like a judgment on who you are, not just what you think, and that blurring of boundaries makes everything feel a lot more personal.

In real life, arguments have built-in limits. Facial expressions, tone of voice, and body language help soften misunderstandings. You can tell when someone's joking, backpedaling, or even feeling hurt. Online? All those social cues vanish, leaving words open to interpretation—and misinterpretation. What might be a harmless snarky joke face-to-face can feel like a direct attack when flattened into black-and-white text.

And because digital arguments lack immediate consequences, people say things they never would in person. There's no awkward silence, no side-eye from mutual friends, no real-time discomfort—just a screen and a sense of emotional distance. This detachment makes it easier to escalate a disagreement, turning minor misunderstandings into full-blown digital warfare.

But the emotional fallout is far from distant. Your brain doesn't distinguish between a real-life threat and a perceived digital one—it simply reacts. When someone challenges your beliefs online, your amygdala (the part of your brain responsible for emotional responses) fires up, flooding your body with stress hormones. Your heart races, your breathing quickens, and you feel an overwhelming urge to clap back—not because it's productive, but because your brain is in fight mode.

## How Online Anonymity Amplifies Aggression

Behind the safety of a screen, people become bolder—and meaner. Psychologists call this the online disinhibition effect, where the anonymity and lack of face-to-face interaction strip away social norms. When no one knows your real name, there's less risk of personal fallout, making it easier to say things you wouldn't dare say in the real world.

This effect is amplified by the illusion of invisibility. Behind a username or anonymous profile, people feel detached from their words, which lowers empathy and heightens hostility. It's not that everyone online is inherently cruel—it's that the environment encourages impulse over reflection. And when people pile on— whether it's a mob dogpiling a public figure or a passive-aggressive subtweet—it becomes a digital free-for-all, where the goal is no longer to understand but to win.

The worst part? You don't have to be anonymous to feel its effects. Even under your real name, social media can feel like a performance stage, where each argument is an opportunity to prove your worth. The drive to be right—to be seen as smart, moral, or superior—can make you stay in fights that drain your energy and chip away at your peace.

## The Emotional Toll of Participating in Digital Drama

No matter how much we pretend otherwise, online fights hurt. Even when you "win" the argument, you rarely walk away feeling better. Instead, you're left replaying the conversation in your head—crafting comebacks you didn't send and obsessing over how others perceived you. This mental loop isn't just annoying—it's exhausting.

Engaging in digital drama triggers a cortisol spike—the same stress hormone released during a real-life confrontation. Over time, repeated exposure to this kind of emotional friction can lead to burnout, increased anxiety, and even emotional numbness. And the aftershocks linger. Long after you log off, your nervous system remains on edge, making it harder to relax, focus, or find joy in offline life.

More insidiously, digital drama can warp your sense of reality. Constant exposure to conflict skews your perspective, making the world feel more hostile than it actually is. It's easy to believe that everyone is always fighting, especially when conflict is amplified by algorithms designed to prioritize controversy over nuance.

And here's the kicker: you don't even need to engage to feel the impact. Just witnessing digital drama—whether it's a celebrity scandal or a blow-up between mutuals—can stir up feelings of secondhand stress, leaving you tense and emotionally drained.

## How to Disengage from Digital Conflict Cycles

The simplest way to avoid digital drama? Don't engage. But let's be honest—that's easier said than done. When you're invested in an issue (or when someone takes a swipe at you), the pull to respond feels irresistible. So, instead of forcing yourself into a "no-conflict" rule, try reframing your response.

Start by recognizing what's worth your energy. Not every fight is yours to fight, and most internet arguments change nothing. Before engaging, ask: Am I solving a problem, or feeding the fire? If it's the latter, it's probably not worth your time.

Next, set digital boundaries. This could mean muting keywords, unfollowing accounts that stir up negativity, or limiting how much time you spend in conflict-heavy spaces. If a specific platform consistently leaves you feeling drained, it might be time to log off—not permanently, but long enough to reset.

When drama does find you, practice the art of the graceful exit. Not every accusation requires a response. Sometimes, the most powerful move is to simply… not engage. Silence isn't weakness—it's a flex of emotional control. You don't owe anyone your emotional bandwidth, and knowing when to disengage is a sign of personal power.

And finally, ground yourself in real-life connections. Online arguments can feel all-consuming, but they're just a tiny fraction of your actual life. Prioritizing face-to-face relationships helps you maintain perspective—and reminds you that the best conversations, the ones that truly matter, happen beyond the glow of a screen.

# 14

# The Emotional Toll of Scrolling

ONE MINUTE, YOU'RE SCROLLING "just for five minutes," and the next, it's two hours later—you're emotionally drained, your head feels foggy, and you can't even remember what you were looking at. That's the social media hangover: the mental and emotional slump that hits after too much time online. Unlike a wild night out, there's no empty bottle to blame—just an endless stream of content that seemed harmless until it wasn't. And yet, despite knowing how terrible it feels, we keep coming back for more.

This isn't just a vibe—it's brain chemistry in action. Every swipe delivers a micro-dose of stimulation, whether it's a funny meme or a heated debate. The problem? Your brain wasn't built for this level of constant input. The more you consume, the more overstimulated your nervous system becomes—leaving you frazzled, depleted, and weirdly numb to both joy and reality. And the crash after a scroll binge? It's not in your head—it's a real, measurable shift in your emotional state.

Social media platforms are designed to keep you hooked— but they're also expert at wearing you out. Each piece of content demands a small slice of your attention, but those slices add up. In the same way your body feels heavy after a junk food binge, your brain feels sluggish after information overload.

And it's not just the volume—it's the emotional whiplash. One second, you're laughing at a pet video. The next, you're reading about climate disasters. Then, a perfectly filtered influencer reminds you that your life doesn't quite measure up. Your brain never gets the chance to process any of it fully, and the constant gear-shifting takes a toll.

Psychologists call this cognitive fatigue—when your mental resources get tapped out from too much input. Scrolling feels easy, but your brain is working overtime behind the scenes, trying to filter, interpret, and react to an avalanche of information. The result? That familiar, post-scroll fog where everything feels too much and not enough all at once.

## The Psychological Crash after Digital Overconsumption

Here's the sneaky part: social media feels energizing while you're doing it, but leaves you drained when you're done. It's a classic dopamine loop—every like, comment, or new post triggers a tiny dopamine hit (your brain's reward chemical). But just like sugar or caffeine, that buzz is short-lived. Once the stimulation stops, dopamine levels dip below baseline, leaving you feeling flat.

This crash is particularly harsh after long, aimless scrolling sessions. When you flood your brain with artificial stimulation, real-life experiences feel dull by comparison. Nothing offline can match the speed, novelty, or intensity of digital content. So, even when you put your phone down, you might feel bored, restless, or emotionally off—not because your life lacks excitement, but because your brain has been overstimulated into exhaustion.

And let's not ignore the emotional residue. The content you consume—whether uplifting or upsetting—doesn't just disappear when you scroll past it. It lingers in your subconscious, creating a low-grade emotional hangover. Maybe it's the lingering unease after doomscrolling through bad news. Or the creeping insecurity after a deep dive into someone else's seemingly perfect life. Either way, the effects stay with you long after you close the app.

## Recognizing Signs of Emotional Burnout

So how do you know when you're sliding into **scroll-induced burnout**? It doesn't hit all at once—it creeps up quietly, disguised as everyday tiredness. But there are some tell-tale signs that your brain and emotions are running on empty:

- Emotional numbness: Everything feels "meh," even things you usually enjoy.
- Irritability: You're snappier, more impatient, and easily triggered.
- Mental fog: It's harder to focus, remember things, or make decisions.
- Social fatigue: Even minor interactions feel exhausting.
- Restlessness: You can't sit still without reaching for your phone, even when you're tired.

These aren't just random mood swings—they're the result of prolonged mental overstimulation. Left unchecked, they can spill over into offline life, making you feel perpetually distracted, disconnected, and dissatisfied.

What's worse? Burnout makes you scroll even more. In search of relief, your brain craves the same quick-fix stimulation that caused the problem in the first place—leading to a vicious cycle where you use social media to escape the exhaustion that social media created.

## Recovery Strategies for Post-Scroll Fatigue

The good news? Social media hangovers aren't permanent—but recovering from them requires giving your brain what it's been missing: rest, intention, and a bit of digital detox. Here's how to recalibrate when your nervous system feels fried:

Step off the content treadmill. Cut back on passive scrolling—especially when you're emotionally vulnerable. This doesn't mean quitting cold turkey (let's be real), but swap mindless swiping for active, intentional screen time. Follow accounts that energize, not exhaust, and unfollow anything that drains you.

Give your brain a buffer. Your mind needs time to process what it consumes. Build in digital-free gaps throughout your day—whether that's tech-free mornings, no-scroll lunch breaks, or putting your phone out of reach during downtime. Even 15 minutes of quiet brain time can reset your mental state.

Detox with dopamine-neutral activities. When your dopamine levels are depleted, slow, sensory-rich activities help recalibrate. Think long walks without your phone, journaling your thoughts, or spending time in nature. Anything that engages your senses (without constant novelty) allows your nervous system to reset.

Check your emotional baggage. Notice how you feel after scrolling. Are you energized? Or low-key drained? Keep a mental note of which platforms and accounts boost or sap your energy—and curate your feed accordingly. If something consistently leaves you feeling worse, that's your cue to mute or block.

Prioritize real-world stimulation. Social media thrives on manufactured experiences, but your brain craves real ones. Prioritize offline activities that nourish your senses—whether that's grabbing coffee with a friend, starting a creative hobby, or simply sitting in the sun. The more grounded in reality you feel, the less tempting the endless scroll becomes.

Ultimately, the best way to dodge the social media hangover is to consume with intention. When you treat your attention like the precious resource it is, you stop feeding the machine that's been draining you dry—and start reclaiming the energy that's rightfully yours.

# 15

# Why You Keep Coming Back

EVER WONDER WHY YOU CAN'T resist checking your phone after posting something—no matter how casual? That itch to see who liked your latest photo or commented on your thoughts isn't just curiosity—it's science-backed addiction, packaged neatly by the world's most powerful tech companies. Every ping, heart, and "omg same" taps into something much deeper than surface-level engagement. It's a carefully crafted cycle of expectation, reward, and craving, and whether you're aware of it or not, it's rewiring how your brain seeks validation.

At the center of this loop is dopamine, the brain's feel-good neurotransmitter. But here's the thing people get wrong—dopamine isn't just about pleasure. It's about anticipation. The moment you post something, your brain flips into a hyper-alert state, waiting for incoming validation. Each like, share, or reply delivers a small but potent dopamine hit—but the real magic lies in the unpredictability of it. If you knew exactly how much attention your post would get, the thrill would disappear. It's the what if factor that keeps your brain hooked. What if the post goes viral? What if someone unexpected reacts? What if you're about to blow up? This uncertainty drives you to check, recheck, and spiral into a dopamine-fueled feedback chase.

Social media platforms know this—and they exploit it

relentlessly. Your notifications aren't delivered all at once by accident. They drip-feed them to you, keeping the cycle alive. The moment you feel like nothing else is happening, another alert pops up. And when it doesn't? That silence isn't just disappointing— it registers in your brain as social rejection. The brain treats being ignored in digital spaces the same way it would treat being shunned from a community back in our hunter-gatherer days. No wonder the absence of likes feels so personal.

And it's not just positive feedback that keeps you locked in. If likes and compliments are the carrot, negative feedback is the stick—and it's even more powerful. A hundred positive reactions can fade into the background, but one passive-aggressive comment? That sticks to your brain like glue. This is because your brain is wired to prioritize threat detection. Back when survival meant watching for predators, paying extra attention to danger kept us alive. Today, that instinct translates to fixating on criticism, even when it comes from a stranger with an anonymous username. And so, the feedback loop isn't just a feel-good mechanism—it's a survival reflex that the internet has turned against you.

What's even sneakier is how personal it all feels. Your social media profiles aren't just platforms—they're extensions of your identity. Every post is a version of you, carefully curated for public consumption. So when the feedback pours in, it's not just a comment on your content—it's a comment on who you are. This emotional entanglement is exactly what platforms want. The deeper you feel connected to your digital persona, the harder it is to step away. It's no longer about casual scrolling—it's about protecting and maintaining an identity that's constantly being shaped by external reactions.

The loop doesn't just capture your attention—it starts shaping your self-worth. Over time, you begin to measure your value by how much engagement you get. Good day? Triple-digit likes. Bad day? Crickets. And because the internet never sleeps, you're caught in an ongoing performance cycle—always presenting, always checking, always craving reassurance. This external validation trap leaves little room for internal confidence. When your sense of self depends on others' reactions, your autonomy shrinks. You're no longer just living—you're performing for feedback.

And don't be fooled into thinking you have full agency here. Algorithms have become disturbingly skilled at understanding what grabs your attention—and they're not neutral. The content you see (or don't see) is designed to provoke an emotional response that keeps you engaged. Ever notice how posts with the most intense reactions—whether outrage, awe, or thirst—tend to flood your feed? That's by design. Platforms prioritize content that fuels emotional highs and lows because it's the emotional charge that keeps you locked into the loop. The more you react, the more valuable you become. Your attention is the product, and algorithms are the salespeople.

And let's talk about the phantom check—that moment when you instinctively reach for your phone even when no notification is there. This isn't random; it's the byproduct of a brain conditioned by years of feedback cycles. The mere possibility of new attention triggers the impulse to check. You're not checking for entertainment—you're checking for affirmation. And the scary part? You probably don't even notice how often you do it. This constant seeking is no longer a conscious choice—it's a habit loop wired into your neurological circuitry.

So how do you break out? The first step is realizing that you're not the problem—the system is. Tech platforms are designed to exploit your psychology, not empower you. Once you see that, you can start untangling your self-worth from digital feedback. One simple but powerful move? Interrupt the loop. When you post something, resist the urge to check immediately. Give your brain space to breathe before the dopamine trap kicks in. Each time you delay that first check, you loosen the loop's grip.

And here's a bold truth: real-life validation hits different. Nothing you post can replicate the feeling of someone seeing and appreciating you in person. When you shift your attention to offline spaces, you start building a self-worth that isn't dependent on push notifications. This doesn't mean deleting your accounts— it means reclaiming control. Platforms might try to shape your emotional world, but your real life is where your worth actually lives.

At the end of the day, the feedback loop isn't just about what the world thinks of you—it's about what you think of yourself when no one's watching. And that's the only validation that really matters.

# 16

# Phantom Buzzes & Fake Urgency

YOU'VE FELT IT BEFORE—YOUR PHONE isn't buzzing, but somehow, you *swear* it did. Maybe it's a phantom vibration in your pocket or a fleeting itch to check your screen. You tell yourself you'll stop—right after you check one more time. And before you know it, you're knee-deep in a group chat you didn't even want to open, and the day slips through your fingers in a haze of notifications that never stop.

This isn't random, and it's definitely not just you. The constant pull toward your phone isn't an accident—it's engineered. Tech companies are in the business of stealing your attention, and one of their best tricks? Making sure you feel like you *can't* afford to miss a thing. And when your brain believes that everything is urgent, unplugging feels like falling behind.

But here's the truth: not everything deserves your attention. And that buzzing feeling? It's not always real. It's a symptom—a side effect of a world where urgency is manufactured to keep you hooked.

Phantom vibrations sound like a weird glitch, but they're so common that there's actual science behind them. Researchers call it "phantom vibration syndrome," and nearly **90%** of people report feeling these fake notifications. It's your brain, rewired by years of digital conditioning, mistaking everyday sensations for something urgent.

Here's what's happening: every time your phone buzzes, your brain releases a hit of dopamine—a chemical tied to pleasure and reward. But the tricky thing about dopamine? It doesn't just show up when you get a reward; it spikes in *anticipation* of one. Your brain has learned to expect a reward (a notification, a message, a like), so it scans for signs constantly—so much so that it starts making up those signals.

It's not just a harmless quirk—it's a red flag. When your brain is constantly on edge, waiting for the next digital dopamine drip, your focus suffers. Instead of being present in the moment, your attention gets hijacked by imaginary alerts. And when you're locked into this cycle, even silence feels loud.

## When Everything Feels Urgent (But Isn't)

Urgency is addictive. That's why social media, messaging apps, and email platforms love it. They use bold fonts, red dots, and push notifications to convince you that *everything* needs your attention right now.

It's called "intermittent reinforcement"—a psychological trick that plays on unpredictability. Sometimes when you check your phone, there's something exciting: a text from your crush, a comment on your latest post, or breaking news. Other times? Nothing. But because you never know which it will be, your brain stays on high alert. And that unpredictability keeps you checking—over and over again.

Apps use this against you. Instagram will delay some notifications so you see them all at once—because a cluster of likes feels more rewarding. TikTok curates random viral videos into your feed to keep you wondering, *What's next?* Even email platforms now "bundle" messages to create an illusion of urgency—because you're more likely to click if you think you're behind.

And this fake urgency has real consequences. It's why you feel stressed, even when nothing important is happening. It's why your focus shatters every time your phone pings. And it's why, no matter how much time you spend online, it never feels like *enough*.

## The Fear of Missing Out (FOMO)—A Digital Weapon

Let's be honest—no one wants to feel out of the loop. And platforms know this. FOMO isn't just a buzzword; it's a psychological pressure point that tech companies exploit. When you're scrolling, there's always a hint of, *What if I miss something important?*

That fear is carefully cultivated. Instagram Stories, Snapchat streaks, and Twitter's trending topics are all designed to feel temporary—if you don't check now, you lose your chance. The algorithm feeds you "what's hot" because nothing feels worse than realizing you missed a viral moment everyone else is already over.

And FOMO isn't just about social updates—it's financial too. Ever felt a rush when a product is labeled "limited time only"? That's intentional. Scarcity makes things seem valuable. So whether it's a limited-drop sneaker or an Instagram Live that disappears in 24 hours, the message is clear: **if you're not paying attention, you're losing out.**

The truth? Most of it isn't that urgent. Your friend's weekend brunch? Still cute tomorrow. That influencer rant? Probably not life-changing. But tech companies don't want you to think like that. They want you to stay hooked—because every second you spend online translates to profit.

## Breaking the Phantom Notification Cycle

So, how do you break free from fake urgency and reclaim your focus? It's not about quitting tech altogether—but it *is* about reclaiming your brain from algorithms designed to exploit it.

Not all notifications deserve your attention. Turn off the non-essentials—especially from apps that thrive on your FOMO. You don't need a ping every time someone likes your photo. When you catch yourself reaching for your phone automatically, pause. Ask yourself: *What am I expecting to find?* Often, the answer isn't something urgent—it's just habit.

Instead of constantly checking throughout the day, set dedicated "check-in" times. This disrupts the dopamine loop and puts *you* in charge of when you engage. Newsflash—you don't need to see everything. Give yourself permission to let things pass you by. The world won't end if you skip a trending topic. Treat your focus like a limited resource—because it is. When you prioritize real-life presence over digital noise, your brain starts to calm down.

Living in a world of phantom buzzes and fake urgency means fighting a system designed to keep you hooked. But the most radical thing you can do? **Unplug on your own terms.**

You don't need to quit social media or throw your phone in a lake. But you *can* choose how and when to engage. You can silence the noise, reject the urgency, and give your brain the peace it craves.

And when you do? That buzzing feeling—the one that keeps you checking—starts to fade. You remember that not everything is urgent, and most things can wait. And the best part? You get your attention back. And in a world built to distract you, that might be the biggest flex of all.

PART 3

Why It's So Hard to Stop

# 17

# The Science of Addiction (And How Tech Exploits It)

YOU TELL YOURSELF YOU'LL ONLY check your phone for a second. Just a quick peek. And yet, an hour later, you're still scrolling, watching, clicking—like a moth to a digital flame. You're not even sure how you got here.

It's not a lack of willpower. It's not a personal failing. It's science—addiction science, to be exact. And tech companies? They know *exactly* how to use it against you.

Digital addiction isn't some exaggerated buzzword—it's real, measurable, and deeply embedded in the way our devices and apps are designed. Social media, endless scrolling, autoplay videos—these aren't just convenient; they're calculated. The same psychological triggers that fuel gambling addiction, binge-eating, and substance abuse are at play in your daily screen habits. And the deeper you go, the harder it becomes to stop.

So, what's happening inside your brain? And more importantly, *how do you break free?*

Here's how tech uses the same principles as gambling. Ever wondered why slot machines are so addictive? You pull the lever, and sometimes you win—sometimes you don't. But the *maybe* is what keeps you coming back. It's called variable reinforcement, and it's the most powerful addiction mechanism there is.

Social media and online platforms run on this exact principle. Every time you open an app, you don't know what you'll get. A new message? A viral post? A flood of likes? Maybe nothing. But that *maybe* is what keeps you checking. Over and over.

Even simple things—like Instagram refreshing your feed with a swipe—are modeled after slot machines. That little delay before new posts appear? That's not lag. That's intentional suspense. Your brain anticipates a reward, gets a dopamine spike from the expectation, and boom—you're hooked before you even realize it.

And it's not just social media. Every "Like," every notification, every unpredictable dopamine hit is designed to make you chase the next one.

## The Neurological Patterns of Digital Addiction

Let's get into the science.

When you engage with digital platforms, your dopamine system—the part of your brain responsible for pleasure and reward—goes into overdrive. Every time you get a new notification, a funny meme, or an exciting update, your brain releases dopamine. And dopamine is what fuels habit formation.

Here's the scary part: your brain *adjusts* to this constant stimulation. The more you indulge, the more you need to feel the same level of reward. It's why scrolling feels satisfying in the moment but leaves you restless afterward. Your brain gets overstimulated and craves *more*.

Over time, this rewiring changes your relationship with technology. You start checking your phone not because you want to, but because your brain expects it. Your focus fragments. Your impulse control weakens. You become *dependent* on the next hit of digital stimulation.

Sound familiar? It should—because this is the same neurological process that fuels drug and gambling addictions.

## Why Your Brain Struggles with Self-Control Online

You might be thinking: *If I know this is happening, why can't I just stop?*

Because your prefrontal cortex—the part of your brain responsible for self-control—is fighting an uphill battle.

Dopamine-driven habits are automatic. They bypass the rational parts of your brain. This is why you find yourself mindlessly opening Instagram before you even *realize* you've done it. It's why TikTok's "one more video" turns into a two-hour spiral.

Tech companies bet on this. They know that impulse control takes effort—and that effort weakens when you're tired, bored, or emotionally drained. That's why social media is most tempting late at night, when your brain is exhausted and your decision-making skills are at their weakest.

And let's be real—tech is convenient. It's easier to escape into digital comfort than to fight your cravings. Your brain *wants* the easy dopamine.

But convenience is a trap. And if you don't recognize how deeply tech is wired into your habits, you'll keep getting pulled back in—over and over again.

## Reversing the Brain's Reward Hijacking

So, is there a way out? Yes. But it's not about quitting cold turkey. It's about rewiring your reward system.

Right now, your brain expects fast, digital dopamine hits. You have to replace that with something more sustainable.

Delay your first check-in of the day. The first thing you do in the morning sets the tone for your brain. If you check your phone first thing, you're priming yourself for distraction all day. Instead, wait at least 30 minutes before opening any apps. Let your brain wake up on *your* terms.

Make dopamine harder to access. Right now, you can get a dopamine hit in seconds. That's the problem. Put barriers in place—move social media apps off your home screen, turn off autoplay, or set timers. When dopamine isn't instant, your cravings weaken.

Retrain your brain with real-life rewards. Tech gives you fake rewards—likes, views, temporary validation. You need real ones. Exercise, deep conversations, creative hobbies—these create dopamine, too, but in a way that fuels long-term satisfaction instead of short-term addiction.

Recognize the urge—then wait. When you feel the impulse to check your phone, pause. Don't fight it, just observe it. Most urges pass within 90 seconds if you don't act on them. Give your brain time to break the cycle.

Rebuild your attention span. Digital addiction destroys focus. Rebuild it with "dopamine fasting." Spend an hour daily on zero digital stimulation—no scrolling, no music, no screens. Your brain will fight it at first, but over time, you'll regain control over your attention.

Right now, tech companies own your brain's reward system. They decide when you get dopamine, how much you get, and what you do to chase it.

But you don't have to play by their rules.

You can take back control. You can *choose* what actually deserves your attention. You can break the cycle.

Because in a world built to keep you addicted, reclaiming your focus is a radical act.

And that's the kind of power no algorithm can steal.

# 18

# Why Your Brain Loves Novelty (Even When It's Trash)

YOUR BRAIN IS A THRILL-SEEKER. Not in a jump-out-of-planes or climb-a-mountain kind of way—but in the quiet, relentless hunger for something new. It's why you refresh your feed the second you feel bored. Why a random TikTok at 2 a.m. feels like a reward. Why you'll click on something, anything, just to feel that tiny spark of interest again. Novelty is the brain's favorite drug, and the internet? It's an endless supply.

At its core, your brain is wired to chase what's new. Evolution designed it that way—when you're scanning for unfamiliar sights or changes in your environment, you're more likely to survive. Back when the most exciting thing around was a rustling bush (could be food, could be danger), this curiosity was a superpower. Fast-forward to now, and that same curiosity is what makes you binge-watch six hours of Instagram reels while your to-do list collects dust.

The internet is like a carnival that never closes. Every scroll, every click, every shiny new notification taps into the brain's obsession with the unfamiliar. But here's the twist: this constant flood of novelty isn't making you happier, smarter, or more fulfilled. It's just keeping you hooked—and exhausted. And the worst part? The more you consume, the harder it gets to stop.

## The Brain's Reward System: Hijacked

Here's the science bit—but don't worry, it's not boring. At the heart of your brain's love affair with novelty is dopamine. You've heard of it—the "feel-good" chemical that's involved in pleasure and reward. What most people don't realize is that dopamine isn't really about enjoyment. It's about anticipation. It's the chemical that fires up when you think something exciting is about to happen, not when it actually does.

Every time you stumble on something new—a funny meme, a breaking news alert, a tweet that makes you furious—your brain releases a little dopamine hit. And that hit feels good. But the real kicker? It feels even better before you click. That moment of *what if*—that's the hook. The internet is built on this exact mechanism. It doesn't just offer content; it dangles it in front of you like a shiny object, promising that the next click might finally deliver what you're craving.

But it never does, not really. Because the brain's novelty circuit doesn't care about satisfaction—it just wants to keep hunting. That's why one video turns into ten. One refresh leads to another. It's not because you're weak-willed—it's because your brain is following an ancient program, one that the modern internet is exploiting to perfection.

## Why We Crave the New (Even When It's Trash)

You've probably noticed that most of what you consume online isn't life-changing. It's quick, disposable, and often, well… garbage. So why can't you stop? The answer lies in how your brain processes novelty.

Novelty signals "importance" to your brain. When you

encounter something new, your brain assumes it matters—even if it doesn't. This is why a random celebrity feud feels urgent or why you can't resist clicking on a headline that promises *you won't believe what happens next*. The brain interprets the unfamiliar as valuable information, even when it's just noise.

And the thing is, the internet is an infinite novelty machine. Algorithms are designed to flood you with fresh content, not because it's good, but because it's new. That's how you end up consuming hours of content you didn't even care about five minutes ago. It's not your fault—it's a design feature.

But here's the dangerous part: the more novelty you consume, the harder it gets for your brain to appreciate slower, deeper forms of reward. A long conversation, a thoughtful book, a quiet moment of reflection—these things can feel… dull. Not because they are, but because your brain has been trained to crave the next shiny thing. And when you're stuck in that loop, everything else starts to feel boring by comparison.

## The Cognitive Cost of Constant Novelty

It's not just your time that's being drained by the endless pursuit of newness—it's your brain's capacity to focus, reflect, and think deeply. Every time you jump from one piece of content to the next, your brain has to reset. This constant switching taxes your cognitive resources. It's called "attention residue"—the mental hangover you get when you never fully disengage from one thing before diving into the next.

And it adds up. Studies show that people who are constantly exposed to rapid, fragmented content struggle with sustained focus. Your ability to process complex information weakens. Your working memory—how much you can hold in your mind at once—shrinks. In other words, the more you snack on mental junk food, the harder it gets to sit down and enjoy a proper meal.

Even worse? This constant flood of new information tricks your brain into feeling busy, without actually being productive. It's why you can spend hours online and still feel like you haven't accomplished anything. Because you haven't. You've just been spinning the novelty wheel, hoping it lands on something that feels meaningful.

## How to Rewire Your Brain for Better Rewards

Here's the truth: breaking free from the novelty trap isn't about quitting the internet or swearing off social media forever. That's not realistic. It's about retraining your brain to crave better rewards—ones that last longer than a five-second dopamine hit.

First, you need to interrupt the autopilot. Most of your novelty-seeking happens without conscious thought. You pick up your phone, open an app, and suddenly, you're three hours deep into TikTok. The key is to create friction—make it harder to mindlessly scroll. Delete the apps you compulsively check. Set intentional "scrolling windows" instead of dipping in and out all day. And when you feel the urge to refresh? Pause. Ask yourself: *What am I actually looking for?*

Second, reintroduce slower pleasures. Your brain didn't always need rapid-fire stimulation to feel satisfied—it learned that habit. And it can unlearn it, too. Start small: read a physical book. Go for a walk without your phone. Call a friend instead of texting. These activities might feel boring at first—that's withdrawal. Push through it. The more you practice, the easier it gets.

Finally, redefine novelty. Not all newness is bad—curiosity is a powerful, beautiful thing. But instead of feeding it with clickbait and outrage, channel it toward something richer. Learn a skill. Dive deep into a topic you love. Let your curiosity stretch beyond the algorithm's limits. Real novelty—the kind that sticks—comes from discovery, not distraction.

The internet isn't going to stop serving up endless junk anytime soon. But you don't have to keep eating it. Your brain deserves better. And with a little intention, you can give it exactly that.

# 19

# The Illusion of Choice

IN A WORLD WHERE EVERYTHING is just a click away, it's easy to believe you're in control. You choose what to watch, which articles to read, and whose lives to scroll through. Or at least, that's how it feels. But beneath the surface of your seemingly independent decisions lies a carefully engineered system—one that shapes what you see, when you see it, and even how you feel about it. The illusion of choice is one of the internet's most sophisticated tricks, and chances are, you've been falling for it without even realizing.

When you open your favorite app, it feels like you're stepping into an endless buffet of possibilities. But the truth is, that buffet has been curated for you—and not necessarily for your benefit. Algorithms, invisible and ever-present, are the ultimate decision-makers. They analyze your habits, track your clicks, and predict what you'll engage with next. It's not just a matter of what's popular; it's about what will keep *you* on the platform for as long as possible. And while it might feel like you're the one making choices, those decisions have already been nudged—sometimes so subtly you don't even notice.

## When Personalization becomes a Trap

At first glance, personalization sounds like a gift. Who wouldn't want a digital world tailored to their interests? Recommendations that know your taste, content that aligns with your views—it all seems like a win. But the problem with this hyper-curated reality is that it's inherently limited. You aren't actually seeing *everything*. You're seeing a version of the world that algorithms think will keep you most engaged.

Take your social media feed. Out of the millions of posts shared daily, you only see a tiny fraction. Algorithms decide which ones make the cut based on an intricate matrix of factors—how long you lingered on a similar post, what you liked last week, even the time of day you're most active. Over time, this creates a bubble where everything feels familiar and comfortable. You start to mistake this limited view for reality, even though there's a vast amount of content that never makes it to your screen.

And it's not just social media. Streaming services, search engines, and even online stores all use similar systems to shape your digital experience. Ever wondered why your Netflix recommendations feel eerily accurate? That's no accident. Every choice you make feeds back into the algorithm, which refines its predictions to keep you watching. The same happens when you search for information—Google's results are not some objective truth; they're a reflection of what the algorithm believes you want to see. And that means two people searching the same term might see completely different realities.

This curated reality has a subtle but profound impact on how you think. When you're only exposed to content that aligns with your interests or beliefs, your worldview narrows. You stop encountering opposing perspectives, which makes your existing views feel more valid and less questioned. This phenomenon, often called the "filter bubble," is why it's so easy to fall into ideological echo chambers online. You're not actively choosing to block out other viewpoints—the algorithm is doing it for you.

## The Myth of Free Will in the Digital Age

It's tempting to believe that you're immune to these influences—that no algorithm can really control your decisions. But the truth is, even the most aware among us are susceptible to digital nudges. Behavioral scientists have found that people make many of their decisions unconsciously, relying on mental shortcuts instead of rational analysis. And digital platforms are designed to exploit those shortcuts.

Consider how effortlessly you fall into the loop of endless scrolling. You didn't actively *choose* to spend two hours on TikTok—you opened the app for a quick distraction, and the algorithm took care of the rest. Auto-play keeps the videos rolling. Personalized recommendations ensure there's always "just one more" to watch. The more you engage, the better the system understands your preferences, and the harder it becomes to break free.

Even the design of digital platforms is built to override your autonomy. The placement of buttons, the color of notifications, the timing of alerts—all of it is engineered to capture and hold your attention. This manipulation isn't random; it's rooted in psychological research that understands exactly how to trigger your brain's reward system. Your curiosity, your need for validation, even your fear of missing out (FOMO)—all of these natural human tendencies are systematically used against you.

This illusion of free will extends beyond what you consume to how you behave. Algorithms don't just predict your actions—they can also shape them. Studies show that subtle changes in how options are presented can dramatically influence your choices. For instance, people are more likely to click on headlines that provoke outrage or curiosity. Platforms know this, which is why your feed is often filled with content that sparks strong emotional reactions. You think you're choosing to engage, but in reality, you're responding to a system designed to make that choice for you.

## Taking Back Control in Digital Spaces

So, if algorithms are constantly shaping your decisions, is it even possible to reclaim your autonomy? The answer isn't to unplug completely—let's be honest, that's neither practical nor desirable in today's world. Instead, the key lies in becoming a more conscious participant in your digital life.

One of the most powerful tools you have is awareness. When you recognize how platforms manipulate your choices, you can start to push back. Ask yourself: *Why am I seeing this?* Most platforms offer some transparency—take advantage of that. On social media, you can often view why a particular ad or post was shown to you. Understanding the mechanisms behind your feed gives you a clearer picture of how curated your experience really is.

You can also disrupt the algorithm's influence by being intentional with your digital habits. Seek out content that challenges your perspective instead of passively accepting what's presented. If you always read the same news outlets, diversify your sources. If your recommendations feel repetitive, search for something new. These small acts of defiance help break the algorithmic loop and expose you to a broader, more authentic range of information.

Another effective strategy is to reclaim your attention. Turn off non-essential notifications. Limit the time you spend on algorithm-driven platforms and set boundaries around your digital consumption. Consider using tools that track your online behavior—seeing how much time you actually spend scrolling can be a wake-up call. And when you engage with content, do it mindfully. Instead of being pulled into an endless stream of recommendations, choose what you consume with intention.

Finally, remember that the most powerful choice you have is where you direct your attention. The internet may be engineered to shape your decisions, but your awareness and intention can still cut through the noise. By actively questioning what you see and reclaiming your digital habits, you can break free from the illusion of choice and take back control of your digital life.

In a world where algorithms dictate so much of what you experience, real freedom comes from the choices you make when you're fully aware of the forces shaping them. And that kind of freedom? It's still yours for the taking.

# 20

# Digital Fatigue

THERE'S A POINT WHERE THE endless stream of content stops feeling entertaining and starts to feel exhausting. You know the feeling—mindlessly scrolling through videos you barely care about, opening new tabs just to close them again, refreshing feeds that never seem to end. It's not boredom exactly. It's something heavier. A kind of mental exhaustion that lingers long after you've put your phone down. Welcome to digital fatigue—a modern-day burnout that isn't caused by work or physical exertion, but by the sheer weight of constant digital stimulation.

At first glance, it doesn't seem like consuming content should be tiring. After all, watching a TikTok or skimming a headline takes mere seconds. But it's not just about the time—it's about what happens to your brain when it's bombarded by information without a break. The human brain is built for complexity, but it wasn't designed to process a never-ending cascade of news alerts, viral trends, heated debates, and meme culture all at once. Eventually, the mental circuits start to overload, leaving you drained, irritable, and craving quiet—but unsure how to actually get there.

Think of your brain like a computer. Every piece of content you consume—whether it's a tweet, a video, or a news article—acts like an open browser tab. One or two tabs? No problem. But when you have fifty tabs running at once, things start to slow down. You lose track of where you started, and eventually, the system crashes. Digital fatigue is the human version of that crash. Your brain is working overtime to process, filter, and make sense of everything it encounters online. And because the content never stops, your mind rarely gets a chance to close those mental tabs and reset.

The nature of digital content makes things worse. Most of it is designed to be fast, shallow, and emotionally charged. Your brain isn't just passively absorbing information—it's making thousands of micro-decisions about whether to engage, dismiss, or store what you're seeing. Is this post funny? Is that headline serious or satire? Should you comment, like, or share? These tiny decisions add up, consuming mental energy without you even realizing. The more content you consume, the more cognitive "bandwidth" you burn through, and the harder it becomes to focus on anything else.

It's no surprise, then, that people who spend more time online report higher levels of mental exhaustion. Studies show that excessive screen time, particularly on social media, can impair memory, attention span, and emotional regulation. What starts as harmless scrolling can quickly become a mental drain, leaving you feeling unfocused and overstimulated. And because digital fatigue often mimics symptoms of general burnout—exhaustion, irritability, and a lack of motivation—it's easy to overlook the real cause: your endless digital consumption.

## When Everything Starts to Feel Meaningless

One of the most insidious effects of digital fatigue is how it erodes your sense of meaning. At its core, your brain craves depth—conversations that matter, stories that stick, experiences that leave an impression. But most digital content is the opposite. It's fast, disposable, and designed to be consumed in rapid succession. Over time, this creates a disconnect. The more surface-level content you consume, the harder it becomes to find meaning in anything deeper.

This is why, after a long session of scrolling, you're often left with a strange sense of emptiness. You've consumed hours' worth of information, yet nothing feels particularly memorable. It's not because your life is boring—it's because your brain has been stuck in a cycle of shallow engagement. Meaning requires reflection, and reflection requires space. When every moment of downtime is filled with digital noise, there's no room left for real thought.

And the fatigue doesn't stop there. Studies on "information overload" suggest that too much digital input can reduce your ability to enjoy offline experiences. When your brain is constantly overstimulated, even simple pleasures—like reading a book, taking a walk, or spending time with friends—can feel less rewarding. It's as if your internal reward system becomes numb. The more you chase digital stimulation, the harder it is to find satisfaction in the real world.

## Signs You're Experiencing Digital Burnout

Recognizing digital fatigue is tricky because it doesn't announce itself the way physical exhaustion does. There's no sudden crash. Instead, it creeps up slowly, manifesting in subtle yet profound ways. You might notice it when:

Your attention span feels shot. Tasks that once felt easy—reading a long article or watching a movie without checking your phone—suddenly seem like a struggle.

You feel mentally drained but don't know why. Even after a full night's sleep, you still wake up feeling sluggish and scattered.

Everything starts to blur together. You can't remember what you saw five minutes ago, let alone yesterday. Content feels repetitive, and nothing holds your attention for long.

You feel restless when you're offline. Downtime feels uncomfortable without a screen to distract you. Silence becomes unfamiliar, even unwelcome.

Your emotions feel blunted. The highs don't feel as high, and the lows don't feel as low. You're stuck in a kind of emotional numbness.

If any of these sound familiar, you're not alone. Digital fatigue is becoming increasingly common in an age where content never stops. But the good news? It's not permanent. With a few intentional shifts, you can reset your mental energy and reclaim your focus.

The antidote to digital fatigue isn't to swear off the internet forever—it's about creating space for your brain to breathe. Here's how to start.

1. **Embrace Digital Minimalism:** Treat your attention as a limited resource. Be ruthless about where you direct it. Unfollow accounts that drain you. Delete apps that no longer serve you. And when you do engage with digital content, prioritize quality over quantity.

2. **Schedule Screen-Free Time:** Your brain needs downtime to process and recharge. Build intentional offline breaks into your day—whether it's a 30-minute walk without your phone or an entire evening spent screen-free. The goal isn't to disconnect permanently; it's to create space for your brain to reset.

3. **Practice Deep Consumption:** Instead of skimming endless headlines, choose one article and read it slowly. Instead of watching ten short videos, engage with a

longer, more meaningful piece of content. Depth is the cure for the shallowness of digital fatigue.

4. **Set Boundaries with Alerts:** Constant notifications fragment your focus and keep your brain in a perpetual state of readiness. Disable non-essential alerts and reclaim control over when—and how—you engage with digital spaces.

5. **Reconnect with Analog Joys:** There's something restorative about tangible, offline experiences. Cook a meal from scratch. Write in a journal. Play a board game. These activities not only give your brain a break but also reconnect you to a slower, more meaningful rhythm.

Digital fatigue is real—but it doesn't have to be permanent. By becoming more intentional about your digital consumption, you can restore your mental energy and rediscover the depth that gets lost in the noise. The internet may be engineered to capture your attention, but your focus? That's still yours to reclaim.

# 21

# Why Deleting Apps
# Isn't a Magic Fix

THERE'S A CERTAIN FANTASY WE all entertain when digital overwhelm hits its peak—the grand app purge. You know the one. You imagine yourself deleting every social media platform, waving goodbye to endless notifications, and suddenly becoming a serene, present version of yourself who reads paperbacks and drinks herbal tea. It's tempting, isn't it? The idea that a single act—deleting the apps—can undo years of digital fatigue and fix your relationship with technology in one bold swipe.

Except, it rarely works that way. If it did, we'd all be living our best unplugged lives by now. But instead, most people who embark on drastic digital detoxes find themselves reinstalling those very same apps within weeks, if not days. The problem isn't just the apps—it's the psychological hold they have on you. And unless you address the deeper reasons you reach for your phone in the first place, no amount of deleting will break the cycle for good.

Here's the thing: apps are designed to be addictive. They're not just passive tools sitting quietly on your phone—they're engineered to trigger powerful psychological responses. Every like, comment, and notification taps into the brain's reward system, delivering tiny hits of dopamine that keep you coming back. So when you delete an app without addressing the underlying craving, your brain doesn't just forget about it. It goes looking for a replacement.

That's why quitting cold turkey often leads to "digital rebound." You might delete Instagram, but soon find yourself obsessively checking email. You uninstall TikTok, only to spend hours doomscrolling news sites. The habit doesn't disappear—it just migrates. And because you haven't tackled the emotional and psychological patterns driving your tech use, the need for constant digital stimulation doesn't go away.

Plus, quitting outright can trigger a subtle but potent form of FOMO (fear of missing out). Social platforms are how many people stay connected—to friends, cultural conversations, and the general pulse of the world. Deleting these apps can create a sense of isolation, leaving you wondering what you're missing. And in moments of boredom or loneliness, the temptation to reinstall and "just check" can become too strong to resist.

## The Psychological Void Left by Digital Withdrawal

It's easy to frame social media as a meaningless distraction, but the truth is, many of us turn to these platforms to fulfill real emotional needs. Connection, validation, entertainment, distraction—apps offer a quick fix for all of these. When you delete them, you don't just lose the content. You lose the coping mechanisms they provide.

Think about it. When you're stressed, what's easier—facing the discomfort or disappearing into a never-ending stream of memes? When you're feeling lonely, is it more tempting to sit with that feeling or scroll through other people's carefully curated lives? Social media, for better or worse, has become the default way many of us process (or avoid) our emotions. And when you strip that away without having healthier alternatives in place, you're left with a psychological void.

This is why many people who attempt drastic digital detoxes experience a form of withdrawal. Anxiety spikes. Boredom feels unbearable. You may even find yourself craving the very platforms you swore off. It's not because you're weak-willed—it's because these apps were filling a psychological gap. And when you remove them, that gap doesn't magically close itself.

## What "Digital Detox" Really Means

The term "digital detox" gets thrown around a lot, but here's the truth: deleting apps isn't the same as healing your relationship with technology. Real digital detox isn't about temporary abstinence—it's about creating lasting balance. And balance requires understanding why you're so hooked in the first place.

A meaningful digital detox doesn't mean swearing off tech forever. It means:

- Identifying the emotional triggers that push you toward endless scrolling.
- Replacing mindless consumption with intentional habits.
- Learning how to engage with digital spaces without letting them consume you.

It's about developing a more conscious relationship with technology—one where you're in control, not the algorithms. This means shifting from automatic habits (like opening Instagram the second you're bored) to deliberate choices about when, why, and how you engage.

## How to Change Your Relationship with Tech (Not Just Quit It)

If deleting apps isn't a magic fix, what actually works? The goal isn't to escape the digital world altogether—it's to engage with it on your own terms. And that starts by rethinking how you interact with technology.

Audit your digital habits. Before you can change your relationship with tech, you need to understand it. Pay attention to how you use different apps. What emotions trigger your scrolling habits? What patterns emerge? Are you reaching for your phone out of boredom, loneliness, or stress? Once you identify the emotional undercurrents, you can begin to disrupt them.

Create intentional boundaries. Instead of deleting apps entirely, try redefining how you use them. Set intentional limits— like only checking social media at specific times of the day or turning off notifications that constantly pull your attention. Consider "single-tasking" online: if you're watching a video, just watch the video. No bouncing between apps. This helps your brain focus and reduces the fragmented attention digital spaces encourage.

Replace, don't just remove. When you delete an app, what fills the void? The key to sustainable change is finding healthier replacements for the emotional needs those apps once met. If you scrolled to relax, find other calming rituals—like reading, meditating, or going for a walk. If you used social media for connection, prioritize face-to-face interactions or phone calls. By giving yourself better options, you reduce the pull to return to old habits.

Practice conscious consumption. Shift your mindset from passive consumption to active engagement. Instead of mindlessly scrolling through endless feeds, ask yourself: What do I want from this? Entertainment? Information? Inspiration? By approaching digital spaces with intention, you reclaim control and make your online time more meaningful.

Embrace digital Sabbaths. You don't need to delete apps to take a break. Designate tech-free periods—an afternoon, a weekend, or even just a few hours before bed. These breaks allow your brain to rest and recalibrate. Over time, you'll notice your mental clarity and emotional resilience improving.

Rebuild your attention span. Constant digital stimulation weakens your ability to focus. Combat this by rebuilding your attention span in small, intentional ways. Start by practicing deep focus activities—reading a book for 20 minutes without interruption or having a conversation without glancing at your phone. These moments of focused presence gradually rewire your brain to resist the lure of constant distraction.

At its core, changing your relationship with technology is about reclaiming your agency. Apps are designed to capture your attention—but you have the power to choose how much you give. Instead of chasing the fantasy of an app-free life, focus on building habits that let you engage with technology in ways that enrich rather than exhaust you. After all, the goal isn't to escape the digital world—it's to exist within it, fully present and in control.

# 22

# Breaking the Habit Loop

IT ALWAYS STARTS THE SAME way—you pick up your phone for something innocent, maybe to check the time or reply to a message. But before you know it, you're knee-deep in a TikTok spiral, eyes glazed over as the minutes bleed into hours. And the wild part? You don't even remember how you got there. It's automatic, like your brain is on autopilot. That's the power of habit loops in action—a cycle of triggers, behaviors, and rewards that keep you coming back, again and again.

The digital world thrives on these loops. Every scroll, tap, and notification feeds into a carefully crafted system designed to hook you. And it works because your brain loves efficiency. Once a behavior is repeated enough times, it becomes automatic— no conscious thought required. So, when you feel a moment of boredom or curiosity, your brain doesn't weigh the options. It just knows: **Open the app. Get the dopamine. Repeat.** And breaking out of this loop isn't as simple as deleting the app. It requires rewiring how you respond to those triggers and finding new ways to satisfy your brain's craving for stimulation.

The science behind habit formation is deceptively simple. It revolves around three key elements: **cue, routine, reward**. First, there's a cue—something that triggers the behavior. This could be an external prompt (like a notification) or an internal one (like boredom or anxiety). Next comes the routine—the behavior itself, whether it's checking Instagram, scrolling through Twitter, or refreshing your inbox. Finally, there's the reward—the dopamine hit you get from seeing something new, funny, or validating. Over time, this loop becomes automatic. You don't even think about it. Your brain just knows that when the cue appears, the reward is a scroll away.

Here's where it gets tricky: tech companies understand this cycle intimately, and they optimize their platforms to keep you locked inside. Infinite scrolls, autoplay features, and unpredictable rewards all play into what's known as **variable reinforcement**—a psychological principle borrowed straight from the world of gambling. When you pull a slot machine lever, you don't know if you'll win, but the possibility keeps you coming back. Social media works the same way. You don't know if the next post will be a hilarious meme, a viral video, or a juicy piece of gossip—but the *chance* that it might be? That's enough to keep you hooked.

What makes breaking tech habits even harder is that these loops often mask deeper emotional needs. You're not just scrolling for fun—you're soothing boredom, numbing stress, or chasing connection. Your phone becomes a convenient escape hatch from uncomfortable feelings. And when you try to quit cold turkey, those unmet emotional needs don't disappear. They sit there, unresolved, pulling you back to the very behaviors you're trying to break.

So, how do you escape a loop that's designed to keep you trapped? It starts with **awareness**. You can't change a habit you don't understand, and most of us operate on digital autopilot. The next time you find yourself reaching for your phone, pause and ask: **What am I feeling right now?** Is it boredom? Stress? Loneliness? Identifying the emotional cue is the first step to disrupting the cycle. Once you recognize your triggers, you can start to **interrupt the pattern**.

Take boredom, for example. If you always turn to social media when you're bored, your brain has learned that scrolling is the quickest path to relief. But boredom itself isn't the problem—it's how you respond to it. Instead of diving into another endless feed, experiment with alternative rewards that satisfy your craving for stimulation without the digital drain. Go for a quick walk, listen to a podcast, or even just sit with the boredom for a moment. The goal isn't to eliminate the cue—you can't always control when boredom strikes—but to **change your automatic response** to it.

This process isn't about willpower; it's about **redesigning your environment** to support new habits. The more friction you create around old behaviors, the easier it becomes to adopt new ones. If you automatically open Instagram first thing in the morning, move the app to a hidden folder—or better yet, delete it from your phone entirely for a while. If late-night scrolling keeps you awake, charge your phone in another room. Small tweaks like these disrupt your usual patterns and make it easier to choose a different path.

At the same time, **building new routines** is crucial. Your brain doesn't like a void—if you remove the habit of scrolling without replacing it with something else, you're more likely to relapse. So, think about what you actually want more of in your life. Maybe it's more face-to-face connection, better sleep, or simply having more mental space. Whatever it is, **anchor new habits** to the moments where you'd normally default to digital distractions. Instead of reaching for your phone during a break, try journaling or stretching. Replace your post-work scroll with a 10-minute walk. The key is to make these new habits both **accessible** and **rewarding**, so your brain begins to associate them with a sense of satisfaction.

And let's be real—there will be moments when you slip back into old loops. That's normal. Breaking deeply ingrained habits isn't about perfection; it's about **persistence**. When you catch yourself falling into the scroll spiral, resist the urge to shame yourself. Instead, treat it as a **data point**—a sign that you still have work to do in understanding your triggers. The more curious and compassionate you are with yourself, the easier it becomes to disrupt the cycle for good.

The most powerful shift you can make is moving from **passive consumption to active choice**. The goal isn't to never touch your phone again—it's to engage with technology **intentionally** rather than by default. When you stop reacting on autopilot, you reclaim your agency. Suddenly, you're not just a passive participant in a habit loop—you're the one in control.

And here's the thing: the more you practice interrupting these patterns, the easier it becomes. Your brain is remarkably adaptable. Every time you choose a new response, you're rewiring neural pathways and weakening the old loops that once held you captive. Over time, those unconscious urges lose their grip, and what once felt automatic becomes a conscious decision. You don't need to quit cold turkey or swear off technology entirely. What you need is the ability to **pause**, to question, and to choose. And once you start exercising that power, you'll realize you've been in charge all along.

# 23

# The Hidden Cost of 'Free' Content

THERE'S A REASON EVERY SOCIAL media platform, streaming service, and news site promises you endless entertainment for the low, low price of... nothing. It sounds like a sweet deal—an infinite buffet of memes, viral videos, and breaking news, all without spending a penny. But here's the twist: you're paying for that "free" content every time you open an app. Not with money—but with your attention, your data, and, ultimately, your mental space. And the real kicker? You're paying a price you probably didn't even realize was on the table.

It's no accident that the most addictive platforms come with no upfront cost. The entire digital economy thrives on attention as currency—and in this system, you're not the customer. You're the product. Every time you scroll, click, or watch, you generate data that's mined, analyzed, and sold. Your online behaviors—the posts you linger on, the videos you replay, even the pauses between swipes—are quietly shaping your digital identity. And while it might feel harmless to give away a bit of personal information for access to free content, the long-term impact is anything but.

The transaction isn't as simple as trading a few data points for a free feed. What you're really giving up is control over your focus. Every moment you spend on a platform is another opportunity for it to capture—and hold—your attention. And they're disturbingly good at it. Tech companies invest billions into understanding how to keep you hooked, using everything from algorithmic predictions to behavioral psychology to craft content that's nearly impossible to resist. The more time you spend glued to a screen, the more valuable you become. Your attention fuels the system, and the system is designed to ensure you never run out of reasons to stay.

But attention isn't the only hidden cost—you're also paying with your mental and emotional bandwidth. The human brain wasn't built to process the sheer volume of information modern platforms hurl at us daily. Yet, here we are, consuming more content in an hour than previous generations encountered in an entire week. And that overconsumption doesn't come without consequences. When your brain is constantly bombarded with new stimuli, it struggles to prioritize what's meaningful. Everything starts to blur together—important insights get drowned out by fluff, and your ability to focus deeply on anything begins to erode.

Over time, this flood of free content subtly shapes how you see the world. Algorithms don't just reflect your interests—they steer them. Every curated feed, recommended video, or trending topic is an invisible hand guiding your perception. And because these systems prioritize engagement over accuracy, the content that rises to the top is often the most sensational, divisive, or emotionally charged. The result? A warped sense of reality where the loudest, most outrageous voices drown out nuance and truth.

The problem is that this shaping happens quietly. You don't wake up one day suddenly believing the world is falling apart—but scroll long enough, and your worldview gradually tilts. You begin to internalize the narratives you're fed, often without realizing that the content you consume has been selected for you, not by you. And because free content is always available, there's no natural stopping point—no built-in moment to pause and reflect. Instead, you're caught in a cycle of endless consumption that leaves little room for critical thought.

The real danger isn't just that free content is persuasive—it's that it's passive. When you let algorithms decide what you see, you're surrendering the ability to choose your own intellectual and emotional diet. And like any diet, consuming whatever's in front of you—without questioning its nutritional value—has long-term effects. Information overload breeds decision fatigue. Your brain, overwhelmed by input, starts to default to easy consumption over active engagement. You lose curiosity. You stop asking questions. And worst of all, you begin to mistake exposure for understanding—as if seeing more content means you know more when, in reality, you're just more saturated.

So, how do you reclaim control in a world where everything is engineered to consume your attention? The first step is awareness—recognizing that "free" isn't free and asking yourself who benefits from your time and energy. When you catch yourself doomscrolling or binge-watching, pause and ask: Is this enriching me, or is it just occupying me? That simple question can snap you out of autopilot and shift you back into a position of conscious choice.

Beyond awareness, it's about cultivating intentional consumption. That doesn't mean cutting yourself off from all digital content—but it does mean being deliberate about what you engage with. Instead of mindlessly accepting whatever algorithms push your way, curate your own intellectual landscape. Follow creators who inspire and challenge you, seek out independent sources that prioritize depth over clicks, and—most importantly—

build in time for offline reflection. Your mind needs space to process and integrate information. Without it, even the most valuable insights slip through the cracks.

And here's the truth: the most valuable things in life often require effort. It's easy to let the digital world serve up endless distractions, but reclaiming your mental autonomy means actively choosing substance over convenience. It means resisting the pull of instant gratification in favor of thoughtful engagement. And while that may feel like swimming against the tide, the payoff is massive. You regain not just your focus, but your capacity for deep thought, real curiosity, and critical awareness—all of which are far too valuable to be traded away for another hour of free entertainment.

Ultimately, shifting from a passive consumer to a conscious user is about more than reclaiming your time—it's about reclaiming your mind. You have the power to decide what deserves your attention. And when you exercise that power, you stop being the product and start becoming the architect of your own experience. Because in a world where attention is the most valuable currency, your ability to choose where you invest it is the ultimate act of freedom.

# 24

# When Screens Steal Your Sleep

THERE'S A MOMENT WHEN THE world quiets down, but your brain doesn't. You're lying in bed, lights off, yet your screen glows bright—a portal to endless content. One more scroll turns into ten, and suddenly, hours have slipped away. By the time you force yourself to stop, sleep feels distant, as if your mind forgot how to switch off. If you've ever felt wired yet exhausted after a late-night binge on your phone, you're not imagining things. Screens are engineered to hold your attention—sometimes at the expense of your rest.

Modern technology isn't just a tool; it's a constant companion. But that companionship comes with a hidden cost. Your brain, a finely tuned biological clock, thrives on rhythm. It expects a natural shift from light to darkness to signal bedtime. But when artificial screens keep flooding your senses late at night, that rhythm falters. The culprit? Blue light. It's the invisible force that tricks your brain into thinking the sun is still up, suppressing melatonin—the hormone responsible for making you sleepy. The later you stare at a screen, the harder it becomes for your body to power down. It's not just a mild inconvenience—it's a biological tug-of-war between your body's need for rest and the artificial world vying for your attention.

But light exposure is only part of the problem. The real

issue lies in what you're consuming. Social feeds are designed to be emotionally stimulating—pulling you into highs, lows, and everything in between. That late-night scroll isn't just visual—it's emotional. The endless loop of news, entertainment, and notifications triggers mental arousal, keeping your brain in a state of heightened activity. And the more emotionally charged the content, the harder it is for your nervous system to unwind. This creates a cycle where your brain stays alert long after your body is craving rest.

The effects go deeper than just feeling tired. Consistently missing quality sleep does more than make mornings harder—it alters how your brain functions. Memory consolidation, emotional regulation, and problem-solving all rely on deep rest. Without it, your cognitive abilities dull. Mood swings become more frequent. Focus slips. Over time, even your immune system weakens, leaving you more vulnerable to stress and illness. What starts as a simple habit—checking your phone before bed—becomes a pattern that can unravel your mental and physical well-being.

What makes screens especially tricky is how they blur the line between being awake and winding down. When your phone serves as both your workplace and your entertainment, there's no clear boundary between activity and rest. Your brain, already overstimulated by a constant influx of digital noise, doesn't recognize when to stop. That's why even when you're physically tired, your mind races—a phenomenon psychologists call sleep procrastination. You know you should sleep, but your brain clings to stimulation, craving one last dopamine hit before letting go.

And then there's the habit loop. Every swipe triggers a reward—a funny video, a new post, an unread message. These tiny dopamine bursts reinforce the behavior, making it harder to quit. Your brain, wired to seek novelty, doesn't naturally want to stop. And when you do finally put the phone down, it's not instant relief. Your mind hums with the leftover noise, making it harder to fall—and stay—asleep.

The kicker? Even when you know screens are interfering with your rest, breaking free isn't easy. Digital habits are deeply ingrained because they're convenient and rewarding. Telling yourself to "just stop scrolling" ignores how these habits hijack your brain's reward circuits. Change happens not by willpower alone but by reshaping the environment and building new rhythms that prioritize rest over endless engagement.

Reclaiming your sleep starts with small, deliberate shifts. It's not about cutting technology out of your life—it's about changing when and how you interact with it. Start by creating a clear transition between your online and offline life. An hour before bed, reduce exposure to screens. This doesn't mean sitting in silence—you can swap scrolling for other forms of unwinding. A physical book, a warm shower, or quiet music can gently cue your brain that the day is winding down.

Your bedroom plays a crucial role, too. Treat it as a screen-free sanctuary rather than an extension of your digital life. Keeping devices out of arm's reach reduces the impulse to check them reflexively. If your phone doubles as an alarm, consider switching to an old-school clock. These small physical barriers disrupt the feedback loop and give your mind permission to settle.

If you still feel tethered to your devices, experiment with nighttime settings that minimize disruption. Most phones now offer "night shift" or "do not disturb" modes, muting unnecessary alerts and reducing blue light exposure. While these features aren't a cure-all, they soften the digital noise, allowing your mind to transition more smoothly into rest mode.

Another powerful shift? Rethink your evening rituals. Instead of seeing sleep as the thing you do after you've exhausted every other distraction treat it as a nightly reset—a way to recharge both your body and mind. Mindfulness practices like deep breathing or gentle stretching can ease mental tension and prepare you for deeper rest. And if your brain still buzzes with unfinished thoughts, consider journaling before bed. Writing down lingering worries gives your mind permission to release them, leaving more room for genuine rest. The truth is, your brain isn't built for constant stimulation. It needs quiet, darkness, and stillness to thrive. And while modern life rarely offers easy exits from digital overload, you have more power than it seems. Prioritizing your rest isn't about rejecting technology altogether—it's about choosing when to step back and allow your mind the break it deserves. At the end of the day—or rather, the night—sleep isn't just a passive state. It's an essential act of self-care. And in a world where screens demand your attention around the clock, protecting your sleep is one of the most radical and restorative things you can do for yourself.

PART 4

Reclaiming Your Mind
(Without Quitting the
Internet)

# 25

# Curating Your Feed (Instead of Letting It Curate You)

WHEN YOU OPEN YOUR FAVORITE social media app, it feels like you're in control. You scroll, you like, you click. But behind every post, video, or suggestion is a carefully engineered system designed to capture your attention and keep you hooked. What shows up in your feed isn't random—it's a reflection of an algorithm's best guess about what will keep you engaged for as long as possible. And while it might feel like you're casually browsing, these seemingly harmless choices shape your thoughts, emotions, and worldview in ways you may not even realize.

The thing is, most of us don't question what we're consuming. We follow people out of habit, curiosity, or obligation, and before we know it, our feeds become a chaotic mix of polished perfection, outrage-driven headlines, and endless distractions. Without realizing it, you're letting algorithms—not your own intentions— shape your mental landscape. And that has real consequences.

Every time you scroll, you absorb information that influences how you think and feel. If your feed is filled with anxiety-inducing news, filtered beauty standards, or performative lifestyles, that content doesn't just stay on your screen. It lingers in your subconscious, quietly shaping your self-perception and mental state. Your mood, your focus, even how you feel about your own life is affected by the digital ecosystem you live in. And when that ecosystem is curated by machines that prioritize profit over your well-being, the cost is deeper than you think.

At its core, the algorithm doesn't care whether what you see makes you feel good, bad, or indifferent—it only cares that you keep scrolling. And it knows exactly how to do that. Emotional content, especially the extreme kind, is more likely to grab your attention. That's why outrage travels faster than joy, why sensationalized stories dominate, and why comparison culture thrives. If you've ever felt emotionally exhausted after an hour of "mindless" scrolling, that's not accidental—it's by design. Your attention is the product, and the algorithm's job is to keep you giving it away.

So, how do you take your power back when the system is built to keep you passive? It starts by becoming an active curator of your digital world. This means rejecting the idea that your feed is an inevitable reflection of the world and realizing you can shape it to serve your mental health and values. You may not be able to rewrite the algorithm, but you can decide what you allow into your mind. And that decision matters.

The first step is to look at your digital consumption with honest curiosity. What are you really feeding your brain every day? Not the content you think you engage with—the content you actually absorb. Pay attention to how your body reacts as you scroll. Do you feel energized or drained? Inspired or insecure? Does a post motivate you to live better, or does it trigger a spiral of self-doubt? It's easy to overlook these emotional shifts because they're subtle—but over time, they add up.

This awareness isn't about judgment—it's about clarity. And once you have it, you can start cleaning house. Think of your feed like your living space. You wouldn't fill your home with things that stress you out or make you feel inadequate, so why do it with your digital environment? Every account you follow either adds to your mental clutter or brings you value. And here's the truth: you don't owe anyone your attention. If a creator, brand, or even someone you know in real life is consistently leaving you feeling worse, you're allowed to unfollow, mute, or block them—without guilt.

Unfollowing doesn't mean you're "too sensitive" or "out of touch"—it means you're taking ownership of what occupies your mental bandwidth. And in a world that constantly demands your attention, protecting your energy isn't just an act of self-care—it's an act of resistance. Algorithms profit from your passivity, but curating your digital space turns that passivity into power.

Curating isn't just about cutting things out—it's also about being intentional about what you invite in. The content you engage with trains the algorithm, which means you have more influence over your feed than you might think. Want to see more of something? Seek it out. Want less of something? Stop engaging with it. Every like, comment, and even how long you hover on a post sends a message about what you want to see. Use that to your advantage.

But curating goes deeper than surface-level preferences. It's also about variety. Algorithms love to trap us in echo chambers where we only see ideas, opinions, and experiences that reinforce what we already believe. And while that's comfortable, it's limiting. Diversifying your feed introduces you to new perspectives, challenges your assumptions, and keeps your mind open. Follow voices that inspire you. Seek out thinkers who challenge you in constructive ways. Find content that stretches your curiosity instead of numbing it.

And don't be afraid to take breaks. Constant consumption, even of good content, can be overwhelming. Our brains aren't built for the endless stream of information that digital spaces provide. Setting intentional boundaries—whether that's limiting your screen time, taking regular social media breaks, or scheduling tech-free hours—gives your mind room to breathe. You don't need to be "plugged in" 24/7 to stay informed or connected. In fact, you'll likely feel more grounded when you're not.

Curating your feed is an ongoing process, not a one-time purge. Algorithms evolve, your interests shift, and your mental needs change over time. Make it a habit to check in with your digital space regularly. Ask yourself: Does this content reflect the life I want to create? Does it support my growth, my peace, and my values? If the answer is no, you know what to do.

The internet isn't going anywhere, and algorithms aren't suddenly going to prioritize your well-being over profit. But within that reality, you still have a choice. You can be a passive consumer, allowing the digital world to shape your inner world without question. Or you can become a conscious curator—someone who chooses what to let in, what to let go, and what to protect.

In a culture where your attention is constantly being hijacked, curating your feed isn't just about what you see—it's about reclaiming your mind. And that is power no algorithm can take from you.

# 26

# How to Stay Aware While Online

YOU TELL YOURSELF YOU'RE JUST going to check one thing—maybe a quick glance at the news, a scroll through your messages, or a peek at social media while waiting for your coffee. And then, twenty minutes disappear. Your thumb moves automatically, your brain hums in the background, and before you know it, you've drifted through an endless stream of content you barely remember consuming. This is the reality of modern scrolling—effortless, addictive, and so routine that it often feels like breathing.

The problem isn't just the time it steals; it's the mental fog it leaves behind. When you scroll without awareness, you're not just absorbing random information—you're handing over your cognitive real estate to whatever the algorithm serves. And because these platforms are designed to hook you, it's frighteningly easy to lose yourself in their pull. What starts as casual browsing quickly morphs into autopilot mode, where your brain disengages, and you simply react to the next thing on your screen.

But here's the thing: you don't have to live at the mercy of your devices. You can scroll with awareness, stay present while online, and reclaim control over your digital habits without quitting cold turkey. Mindful scrolling isn't about demonizing technology—it's about using it on your terms, not theirs. And it begins by recognizing the invisible switch that flips between conscious engagement and mindless consumption.

Your brain loves patterns. When you repeat a behavior enough times—whether it's refreshing an app, checking notifications, or scrolling through TikTok—it becomes automatic. This efficiency is helpful in certain contexts (you don't have to think about tying your shoes every morning), but it works against you when tech platforms exploit it. Scrolling without thinking isn't a personal failing—it's a habit loop engineered to keep you hooked. But the moment you start paying attention to your patterns, you disrupt the loop. And disruption is where change begins.

The first step toward mindful scrolling is to recognize when you slip into autopilot mode. It's surprisingly easy to miss because it feels familiar—your hand moves before your brain even catches up. Pay attention to those reflexive moments. When do you instinctively reach for your phone? Is it when you're bored? Anxious? Procrastinating? Notice the triggers that send you straight to the scroll. Awareness isn't about judgment; it's about observing your habits with curiosity instead of shame.

Once you start spotting your scroll triggers, you can build intentional pauses into your routine. These aren't grand, time-consuming rituals—they're simple mental checkpoints that snap you out of autopilot and back into the present. Before you open an app, pause and ask yourself: "Why am I here?" Is it to check something specific? To connect with someone? Or are you just filling a void? This tiny act of questioning interrupts the automatic urge and invites intention into the equation.

You can also use environmental cues to signal mindfulness. For example, if you always scroll in bed, at your desk, or while watching TV, those settings become linked with unconscious consumption. Shake things up. Scroll in a different space. Hold your phone in your non-dominant hand. Change your lock screen to a reminder—something simple like *"Is this worth my attention?"* These small tweaks break habitual patterns and keep you present.

Another powerful tool? Micro-pauses. These are brief, intentional breaks you insert during your scroll sessions to check in with yourself. After a few minutes of browsing, stop and ask: *How do I feel right now?* Energized? Drained? Inspired? Irritated? This simple practice reconnects you with your emotional state and helps you gauge whether your scrolling is adding value or simply numbing you. It also pulls you out of the algorithm's grip and back into your body—an essential move when tech is designed to disconnect you from physical awareness.

One of the biggest traps of mindless scrolling is its time distortion effect. You think you've been online for five minutes, but when you glance at the clock, half an hour has vanished. To counter this, try intentional timeboxing—set a specific timeframe for digital engagement. Instead of scrolling indefinitely, tell yourself, "I'll browse for ten minutes, then stop." Use a timer if you need to. This isn't about rigid control—it's about creating natural endpoints so your scroll doesn't stretch endlessly.

Mindful scrolling is also about what you consume, not just how you consume it. Algorithms reward extreme content because it generates engagement, but that doesn't mean you have to feed your brain a steady diet of rage bait and clickbait. Curate your digital space with intention. Follow people who inspire you. Seek out voices that expand your thinking rather than narrow it. And when content consistently leaves you feeling anxious, angry, or hollow—mute it, unfollow it, or walk away. Your mental health is more important than staying digitally "in the loop."

Of course, you don't need to be hyper-vigilant every time you touch your phone. Mindful scrolling isn't about perfection—it's about staying awake in a system that thrives on your passivity.

Some days, you'll catch yourself before you spiral into a two-hour doomscroll. Other days, you'll blink and realize you've fallen down another algorithmic rabbit hole. That's okay. The goal isn't to eliminate distraction altogether—it's to develop enough awareness to choose when and how you engage.

And the truth is, mindful scrolling isn't just about saving time. It's about reclaiming your mental space. When you stop operating on autopilot, you free up cognitive energy for things that actually matter—your relationships, your creativity, your peace of mind. You become an active participant in your digital life rather than a passive consumer.

The internet isn't going to slow down. Content will keep multiplying, algorithms will keep optimizing, and the temptation to scroll endlessly will never fully disappear. But your attention is still yours to direct. And by practicing mindful scrolling, you remind yourself—over and over again—that you're in charge.

Because in a world that constantly pulls you toward distraction, choosing awareness is a radical act of self-care.

# 27

# Rewiring Your Brain for Deep Focus

YOUR BRAIN WASN'T BUILT FOR the endless barrage of notifications, open tabs, and dopamine hits disguised as digital updates. Yet, in a world where multitasking is glorified and attention is constantly fragmented, staying focused feels almost impossible. Scrolling while watching TV, checking emails during meetings, or flipping between five different apps at once isn't just a habit—it's a rewiring of how your brain processes information. And it comes at a cost.

When your mind is bombarded by stimuli, it loses the ability to sink into deep focus. That immersive, undistracted state where you can think clearly, work efficiently, and actually *feel* your mind engage? It's getting harder to reach because the digital world thrives on keeping you overstimulated. But here's the truth: no matter how scattered your attention feels right now, your brain is capable of change. Through neuroplasticity—your brain's ability to reorganize and form new neural connections—you can rebuild your capacity for deep focus. But it takes intentional effort to undo the overstimulation and reclaim your mental clarity.

At the heart of this struggle lies your brain's reward system. Every notification, new post, or flashing update gives your brain a micro-dose of dopamine—a neurotransmitter linked to pleasure and motivation. Over time, your brain learns to crave these quick hits, prioritizing novelty over sustained effort. This is why focusing on a single task can feel painfully dull compared to the rapid-fire satisfaction of scrolling. You're not lazy or broken—your brain is simply responding to the digital environment it's been trained in.

The good news? Just as your brain adapts to distraction, it can also relearn how to focus. And while the idea of "detoxing" from tech sounds dramatic, the process of rewiring your brain doesn't require extreme measures. It starts with small, deliberate shifts that teach your mind to value sustained attention again.

One of the most effective ways to begin is by creating intentional "focus sprints"—short, distraction-free periods where you engage deeply with a task. This works because your brain thrives on rhythm and repetition. By carving out even 10-15 minutes for undivided focus, you gently retrain your mind to stay with a task instead of jumping between stimuli. Start small and build gradually—over time, these focused intervals strengthen your brain's ability to resist digital pull and sink into deeper work.

But focus sprints alone won't work if your environment is constantly signaling you to switch tasks. Digital overstimulation doesn't just exhaust your attention—it rewires your brain's baseline state. To counter this, you need to create what cognitive scientists call "attention-friendly environments." This means designing physical and digital spaces that minimize friction and promote flow. Simple changes—like turning off non-essential notifications, using 'Do Not Disturb' during work blocks, and keeping your phone out of arm's reach—can significantly reduce the mental noise pulling at your focus.

Equally important is how you transition between tasks. Each time you switch focus—from a work document to a social media feed to an email—your brain incurs what's known as a "cognitive cost." It takes time and mental energy to recalibrate each time you shift contexts, making your thinking slower and more fragmented. This phenomenon, called "task-switching fatigue," drains your cognitive resources without you even realizing it. The solution? Batch similar tasks together and minimize context-switching. For example, check emails at set times instead of constantly dipping in and out throughout the day.

Another overlooked factor in focus recovery is mental rest. In a world obsessed with productivity, we often undervalue stillness—but your brain needs downtime to function optimally. Research shows that activities like daydreaming, taking nature walks, or engaging in simple, screen-free tasks promote "default mode network" activity—a critical brain state linked to creativity and deep thought. Integrating short, restorative breaks into your day isn't a luxury; it's a necessity if you want to maintain long-term cognitive health.

Training your brain for deep focus also means addressing the emotional component of digital overstimulation. It's not just about willpower—your relationship with focus is deeply tied to how you manage stress and discomfort. Many of us instinctively reach for our phones when we're anxious, bored, or overwhelmed because it offers a quick escape. But true focus requires learning to sit with that discomfort instead of numbing it with distraction. Mindfulness practices—like focused breathing or body scans— can help you develop the mental resilience to stay present when focus feels challenging.

There's also a crucial shift that happens when you redefine focus as a skill rather than a fixed trait. You're not inherently "bad at focusing"—your brain has simply adapted to a fragmented world. When you approach focus as something you can strengthen through practice, you take back agency over your attention. This mindset shift is empowering because it reframes the struggle as something you can work on rather than something you're doomed to accept.

Building this new relationship with focus isn't about perfection. Some days you'll feel sharp and present, while others you'll catch yourself mid-scroll wondering how you got there. That's normal. What matters is consistency—showing up for your focus practices, even when it feels hard. Over time, these small actions accumulate, rewiring your brain for deeper concentration and a more intentional life.

Ultimately, reclaiming deep focus isn't just about productivity. It's about giving yourself the mental space to think, reflect, and be fully present in your own life. In a world that constantly competes for your attention, choosing to direct your focus—rather than letting algorithms do it for you—is an act of self-preservation. You have the power to change how your brain engages with the digital world. And that power starts with reclaiming your focus, one intentional moment at a time.

# 28

# The Power of Pause

EVERYTHING DEMANDS YOUR ATTENTION—BUZZING NOTIFICATIONS, endless feeds, and the pressure to be always "on"—the concept of pausing feels almost radical. Modern life encourages speed, reaction, and constant input. We absorb information faster than our brains can process it, filling every quiet moment with noise. But beneath the surface of this digital hustle something crucial gets lost: mental space. Without pause, there's no room for reflection, clarity, or genuine presence. And when your mind is always occupied, it's easy to mistake constant activity for meaningful engagement.

The human brain isn't designed to process a relentless stream of stimuli without breaks. Every piece of information you encounter—whether it's a tweet, a news headline, or a text message—requires mental energy to interpret and store. When that input never stops, your cognitive system becomes overloaded. It's like running too many apps on your phone at once; eventually, the system slows down or crashes. This cognitive overload doesn't just lead to mental exhaustion—it also blocks the brain's ability to think deeply and regulate emotions.

Pausing isn't just a luxury—it's a biological necessity. Studies show that the brain needs downtime to consolidate memories, process emotions, and make sense of experiences. When you skip these mental breaks, your thoughts become scattered, your emotional regulation weakens, and decision-making becomes less precise. Without intentional pauses, the brain is stuck in reactive mode—constantly responding to external stimuli instead of engaging in reflective, deliberate thinking.

And yet, the digital world is designed to discourage pauses. Social media platforms and news feeds are built on infinite scrolls, intentionally removing natural stopping points. This keeps you in a state of passive consumption, where one post leads to the next without giving your brain a chance to breathe. Even the briefest moments of stillness—waiting in line, sitting at a red light—are filled with the urge to check your phone. But when you never pause, you lose access to deeper cognitive processes like creativity, problem-solving, and emotional insight.

Reclaiming mental space requires breaking this cycle by deliberately inserting pauses into your digital life. These pauses don't have to be dramatic; even brief moments of intentional stillness can reset your brain's rhythm. Psychologists refer to these as "micro-pauses"—short breaks that interrupt the flow of constant input and allow your mind to reset. A micro-pause could be as simple as closing your eyes for 30 seconds, taking a few slow breaths, or stepping away from your screen between tasks. These small moments disrupt the overstimulation loop and give your brain the chance to recalibrate.

The benefits of pausing extend beyond cognitive clarity—they also influence your emotional well-being. Constant exposure to digital content, especially emotionally charged material, keeps your nervous system on high alert. You might not consciously register the impact, but scrolling through distressing news or heated debates activates your brain's stress response. Over time, this low-grade anxiety becomes a background hum, leaving you tense and emotionally depleted. Pausing helps to interrupt this stress cycle by signaling your nervous system to slow down and return to a calm baseline.

One powerful way to harness the benefits of pausing is through the practice of "conscious interruption." This means deliberately stepping out of your habitual digital routines to create moments of stillness. For example, instead of moving straight from one online task to the next, take a 60-second pause to check in with yourself. Ask: How do I feel right now? Is this activity adding value or draining me? These questions may seem simple, but they disrupt autopilot behavior and bring awareness back to your experience.

Pausing also enhances your capacity for emotional regulation—a crucial skill in a world that thrives on reactive behavior. Without space to process your feelings, it's easy to get swept up in digital outrage or anxiety loops. By inserting intentional breaks, you give yourself the opportunity to observe emotional triggers instead of immediately reacting to them. This can be as simple as taking a breath before responding to a heated comment or closing an app when you notice it's heightening your stress. Over time, these small pauses strengthen your ability to respond with intention rather than impulse.

Beyond micro-pauses, larger "macro-pauses" are essential for long-term mental clarity. Macro-pauses are extended breaks from digital input—anything from a tech-free morning to an entire weekend offline. These deeper pauses allow your mind to decompress and reset fully. During these breaks, you may notice a mental shift: thoughts become clearer, your attention stabilizes, and your emotional bandwidth expands. Far from being a retreat from modern life, these pauses provide the mental spaciousness necessary to engage with the world more fully.

The resistance to pausing often comes from a fear of "missing out" or falling behind. In a culture that equates busyness with productivity, stillness can feel like a waste of time. But the truth is, constant motion doesn't equate to meaningful progress. Without mental space, you lose the ability to reflect, prioritize, and make intentional decisions. Pausing isn't about withdrawing from life—it's about creating the conditions to participate in it more fully.

Practicing the power of pause isn't about perfection. Some days, you'll forget to step back. Other times, the urge to stay plugged in will feel stronger than the desire for stillness. That's okay. The point isn't to escape technology but to build a more balanced relationship with it—one where your attention is yours to direct. Every time you pause, you reclaim a small piece of your mental landscape. Over time, these moments accumulate, creating a life that feels less reactive and more intentional.

In the end, the ability to pause isn't just about managing digital overwhelm—it's about reclaiming the most valuable resource you have: your attention. When you choose to pause, even for a moment, you take back control from the systems designed to scatter your focus. And in that space, you rediscover something priceless—your ability to think, feel, and be fully present in your own life.

# 29

## Intentional Consumption

MORE ISN'T ALWAYS BETTER—IT'S OFTEN just louder. Every scroll, click, and tap delivers an endless cascade of information vying for your attention. It's easy to believe you're in control, selecting what to consume, but in reality, much of your digital experience is shaped by algorithms designed to maximize engagement, not your well-being. This creates a constant tug-of-war between your time and the content you consume—one that often leaves you mentally drained rather than informed or inspired. The answer isn't to quit consuming altogether; it's to become a more intentional consumer—one who actively chooses content that enriches, rather than overwhelms, their life.

At its core, intentional consumption is about quality over quantity. Just because content is available doesn't mean it deserves your attention. The internet thrives on abundance—millions of posts, videos, and updates flood your feeds daily. But this overload can leave you feeling scattered and unfocused. Each time you absorb new information, your brain processes it, whether you realize it or not. When you consume mindlessly, that processing power gets wasted on shallow, repetitive, or even harmful content, which diminishes your capacity for deeper thought. The first step toward intentional consumption is recognizing that your mental energy is finite—and treating it like a valuable resource rather than something to squander.

One powerful strategy for curating better content is conducting a digital audit. Take a step back and assess the media you engage with daily. What do you read, watch, and listen to regularly? Does it leave you feeling inspired, informed, or connected? Or does it trigger anxiety, comparison, and fatigue? Pay attention to how your body and mind react after engaging with specific content. If something consistently leaves you feeling worse, it's a signal to reevaluate whether it deserves a place in your digital diet. The goal isn't to shut yourself off from the world but to filter out the noise that drains you while amplifying content that nurtures your mental and emotional health.

One of the biggest traps of unintentional consumption is the illusion of being "informed." We live in an age where news breaks constantly, and the fear of missing out on critical updates can lead to compulsive checking. But being bombarded with headlines doesn't make you better informed—it often just heightens your anxiety. Studies show that overexposure to distressing news can lead to "headline stress disorder," where constant consumption of crisis content leaves you feeling helpless and overwhelmed. A more intentional approach involves limiting your exposure to breaking news cycles while choosing slower, more in-depth journalism that offers context rather than chaos. It's not about turning a blind eye—it's about preserving your mental bandwidth for things that actually matter.

The algorithms that shape your digital world are not neutral. Every platform you engage with—whether it's social media, streaming services, or news sites—relies on algorithms that prioritize content designed to keep you hooked. This means that if you passively consume, you're allowing these systems to decide what you see, think, and feel. Being intentional means taking back control. Unfollow accounts that fuel comparison or negativity. Mute notifications that constantly pull your attention. Follow creators, thinkers, and platforms that align with your values and goals. This doesn't just change your feed—it changes your perspective. When you surround yourself with thoughtful, nourishing content, you cultivate a mindset of growth and curiosity rather than one of constant distraction.

Curating your content diet isn't just about cutting out the bad—it's about actively seeking out the good. Think of your digital consumption like a meal plan: a mix of information, inspiration, and entertainment. Prioritize media that challenges your assumptions, deepens your understanding, or brings you joy. Diversify your sources to include voices and perspectives outside your immediate bubble. This not only protects you from algorithmic echo chambers but also fosters a richer, more nuanced view of the world. A well-rounded content diet doesn't numb your brain—it fuels it.

It's also crucial to establish boundaries around when and how you consume. Without intentional guardrails, content will seep into every corner of your life—interrupting your work, your relationships, and even your rest. Set clear limits around screen time, especially during moments of mental downtime. For instance, resist the urge to scroll during your morning routine or before bed—two times when your brain needs quiet, not noise. Create intentional "off" windows where you step away from screens altogether. This isn't about depriving yourself—it's about creating breathing room for deeper reflection and real-life connection.

Another powerful tool for intentional consumption is practicing digital minimalism. This doesn't mean deleting every app or going full tech-free; instead, it's about keeping only what adds value. Audit your subscriptions and online communities regularly. Are they enhancing your life, or are they just filling space? By pruning what no longer serves you, you make room for content that enriches your thinking and feeds your curiosity. Minimalism isn't about scarcity—it's about making intentional choices that prioritize quality over clutter.

Intentional consumption also means interrogating your motivations. Why are you reaching for your phone? Are you genuinely interested, or are you avoiding discomfort? Many digital habits are driven by emotional triggers—boredom, stress, or loneliness. By recognizing these patterns, you can pause before falling into mindless scrolling. The next time you find yourself on autopilot, ask: "Is this serving me, or am I serving it?" This question disrupts the compulsion and creates space to make a conscious choice.

The beauty of intentional consumption is that it's customizable. There's no one-size-fits-all formula because your needs, interests, and values are unique. What matters is that you remain in the driver's seat. Instead of letting algorithms and external forces dictate your attention, you become the curator of your own mental landscape. This shift doesn't happen overnight—but small, consistent adjustments compound over time. Each intentional choice reclaims a bit of your mental clarity and emotional bandwidth.

In a culture that rewards constant consumption, choosing to be intentional is a radical act of self-care. It's a commitment to honor your attention as something precious rather than giving it away without thought. When you curate your digital environment with care, you're not just shaping what you see—you're shaping how you think, feel, and engage with the world. And in a sea of endless noise, that kind of clarity is a rare and powerful thing.

# 30

# Detox without Disconnecting

THE IDEA OF A FULL digital detox sounds seductive—just unplug everything, toss your phone in a drawer, and reclaim your brain. But reality rarely works that way. In a world where screens are stitched into everything—work, relationships, even how we relax—going cold turkey is often unrealistic and, frankly, unnecessary. The goal isn't to abandon technology altogether; it's to find a healthier balance where your devices work for you, not the other way around. Small, intentional shifts can have a massive impact without forcing you to disconnect entirely. It's about creating breathing room in your digital life while still staying connected to the things that matter.

The problem with quitting cold turkey is that it doesn't address the root cause. Sure, deleting every app might offer temporary relief, but it doesn't change the patterns that got you hooked in the first place. Like any other habit, screen time is deeply intertwined with your emotional landscape—stress, boredom, or even loneliness often trigger the urge to scroll. Without addressing these triggers, you'll likely find yourself reinstalling everything the next time you need a distraction. The more sustainable approach is to focus on small, consistent tweaks that reduce overwhelm without the extremes of a total blackout.

One of the most effective ways to start a tech detox without disconnecting is to create *tech-free zones*. These are physical spaces where screens simply don't belong. Think of them as digital sanctuaries—places where your brain can rest from the constant influx of information. Your bedroom is a great place to start. Keeping devices out of your sleep space improves both the quality of your rest and your mental clarity. Instead of doomscrolling before bed, swap your phone for a book or journaling session. By reclaiming this one area, you give your brain the break it craves while preserving your ability to stay connected elsewhere.

Time-based boundaries work just as powerfully as physical ones. Tech-free windows in your day allow you to reclaim moments of quiet without giving up your devices entirely. Mornings, for example, are prime real estate for a micro-detox. Instead of diving straight into notifications, give yourself the first hour of the day without screens. This small shift sets a calmer tone and allows your thoughts to surface without external noise. Evening wind-downs also benefit from intentional tech breaks— swapping that last-hour scroll for mindful downtime can ease your brain into better sleep. These windows don't have to be long to be effective. Even 20-minute tech-free pockets scattered throughout your day offer a refreshing mental reset.

Another easy, high-impact tweak is *batch-checking*. Constantly checking emails, messages, and social feeds fragments your focus, making it harder to engage deeply with anything. Instead of grazing on notifications all day, carve out specific times to check and respond. This might mean limiting social media to designated windows or only reading emails during work hours. By reducing the frequency of your checks, you protect your attention span while still staying connected. It's not about cutting yourself off—it's about reclaiming control over when and how you engage.

Micro-detoxes—short, intentional breaks from screens—are

another powerful tool. These aren't week-long retreats; they're bite-sized pauses you can weave into your everyday routine. A five-minute walk without your phone. An hour offline during dinner. A weekend afternoon spent reading or outdoors. These moments allow your brain to decompress without requiring a total tech exile. The key is consistency. Regular micro-detoxes give your brain breathing space to process and reset while allowing you to remain digitally present the rest of the time.

One of the most overlooked aspects of digital overwhelm is the clutter. Your phone, laptop, and inbox are often stuffed with apps, subscriptions, and notifications you no longer need but still drain your attention. Digital decluttering is a simple yet effective way to detox without disconnecting. Unsubscribe from newsletters you don't read. Delete apps you only open out of habit. Mute or unfollow accounts that add stress rather than value. Each piece of digital clutter you remove lightens your mental load, making it easier to engage with the things that truly matter.

It's also worth reconsidering *how* you consume content. Mindless scrolling tends to happen when there's no clear intention behind it. Instead of reaching for your phone automatically, try asking yourself: *What am I here for?* Are you looking for entertainment, connection, or information? This small pause can interrupt autopilot mode and guide you toward more mindful consumption. If your current habits aren't serving you, swap them for intentional alternatives—podcasts that inspire, books that challenge you, or conversations that nourish real-world connections.

One powerful reframe is to view your tech habits as something you *design* rather than something that happens to you. You're not at the mercy of your devices—every swipe, click, and tap is a choice. Instead of relying on willpower to avoid distractions, change the environment itself. Keep your most-used distractions out of immediate reach. Use tools like screen time limits, focus modes, and app blockers to enforce the boundaries you set. This isn't about self-denial—it's about curating a digital world that supports your priorities.

Importantly, detoxing without disconnecting isn't a one-size-fits-all formula. What works for someone else may not work for you. The goal isn't perfection—it's progress. Small shifts compound over time. Whether it's taking your lunch break without a screen, silencing notifications during deep work, or designating tech-free evenings, each adjustment helps you reclaim a little more of your mental clarity.

Ultimately, the most sustainable digital detox is one you can live with long-term. Extreme solutions rarely stick because they ignore the realities of modern life. But by integrating small, intentional changes, you can break the cycle of overwhelm while staying connected to the digital world in a way that feels healthy, empowering, and entirely on your terms.

# 31

# Digital Boundaries
# That Actually Work

THE PHRASE *"I'LL SCROLL LESS"* sounds like a good idea—until you find yourself three hours deep into a random influencer's skincare routine. Vague promises like that rarely work because they're based on hope, not a plan. In a world where everything is designed to keep you hooked, *fuzzy intentions* are no match for the relentless pull of endless content. Real digital boundaries—the ones that actually work—aren't about banning screens altogether or relying on willpower. They're about setting specific, flexible rules that fit your life while protecting your mental space. Without clear boundaries, it's easy for the digital world to seep into every crack of your day, blurring the line between *being online* and *being alive.*

Most people fail at setting tech limits because they aim for perfection. You swear you'll stop checking your phone in bed, and by day three, you're refreshing TikTok at midnight like a lab rat hitting a dopamine lever. The secret isn't rigid rules—it's flexible guardrails that work with how your brain and habits actually function. The goal isn't to become a digital monk who's never online. It's about reclaiming your attention, protecting your mental energy, and deciding how you want to engage instead of being on autopilot.

So, where do you even start? Not with grand declarations. You don't need to unplug from life or live in a Wi-Fi-free yurt. Real digital boundaries start with noticing the problem zones— those slippery moments when "just five minutes" becomes two hours. Maybe it's the endless post-work scroll that eats up your evening. Or the way your brain twitches for notifications during every quiet pause. Pinpoint the triggers first. The most effective boundaries are tailored, not generic. If your biggest weakness is doomscrolling before bed, your solution looks different from someone who can't stop refreshing work emails on vacation.

One powerful trick is to externalize the boundaries. Willpower is overrated when you're up against a billion-dollar industry engineered to capture your attention. Don't rely on vague promises to "be better." Instead, use tools to enforce limits. App timers, focus modes, and screen-time locks can act like a personal bouncer between you and the digital vortex. And here's the catch: make the boundary slightly inconvenient to break. If turning off an app lock is too easy, you'll bypass it the moment boredom strikes. But if breaking the rule requires extra steps—like inputting a password you gave to a friend—it forces a moment of reflection. That pause is often enough to snap you out of the automatic scroll.

Another sneaky boundary-breaker? The illusion that "quick checks" don't count. You tell yourself you're just peeking at a notification, but the next thing you know, you've fallen down a Reddit rabbit hole. Those micro-checks are deceptively costly— they fragment your focus and keep your brain in a state of low-grade anxiety. To combat this, create buffer zones—specific times or spaces where tech is off-limits. This isn't about cutting yourself off entirely but giving your mind permission to rest.

Try a "no-phone-first-hour" rule in the morning, or make your bedroom a tech-free sanctuary. It's not about deprivation—it's about reclaiming mental breathing room.

Social pressure is another boundary-wrecker. You know the drill: Someone texts you, and you feel compelled to respond immediately—even when you're exhausted. The modern world runs on instant access, and saying, "I'm offline for a bit," can feel radical. But here's a wild thought: You are not obligated to be digitally available 24/7. Setting expectations with others is a boundary game-changer. Let people know you're not glued to your phone, and normalize delayed responses. The people who truly matter will respect your limits. And anyone who doesn't? That's their problem, not yours.

But what about work? The blurred line between professional and personal life makes digital boundaries extra tricky. If your inbox feels like a never-ending to-do list, it's time to reestablish control. Set specific "off-the-clock" hours where work emails are out of sight. Many people fear that setting these limits makes them seem uncommitted—but the reality is that burnout serves no one. Clear, kind communication is your best tool here. Inform colleagues of your boundaries ("I don't check emails after 7 p.m.") and stick to them. Consistency breeds respect.

Here's another curveball: Boundaries aren't just about **less** time online—they're also about better quality time. Mindless scrolling drains you, but intentional digital consumption can nourish you. Instead of cutting off all tech use, reshape it. Follow accounts that uplift and inform you. Unsubscribe from content that leaves you drained or anxious. Curate a digital space that aligns with who you want to be—not just what the algorithm serves up. This shift transforms screen time from a mindless escape into something that adds genuine value.

And yes, you're allowed to change your boundaries as life evolves. What works during a busy work season might feel restrictive when you're on vacation. Boundaries aren't fixed—they're fluid. Check in with yourself regularly: Is your current digital consumption energizing or exhausting you? If it's the latter, tweak your limits without guilt. Remember, the point isn't to create more rules to follow—it's to craft a relationship with technology that feels empowering instead of depleting.

If you're craving a quick boundary boost, start small. Try a 20-minute "focus sprint" where all distractions are muted. Designate one evening a week as a "screen-free zone" and reconnect with offline pleasures—books, hobbies, or actual human conversation. These micro-boundaries might seem insignificant, but they stack up over time, rewiring your habits in a sustainable way.

The biggest takeaway? Digital boundaries work best when they're rooted in self-respect, not self-denial. You don't need to punish yourself for loving the internet. But you also don't need to let it run your life. The power lies in conscious choice—deciding when, where, and how you engage with digital spaces. Because the internet isn't going anywhere—but you deserve to navigate it on your terms.

# 32

# How to Resist the Next Viral Rabbit Hole

VIRAL CONTENT IS EVERYWHERE—BLARING FROM your phone screen, popping up on social feeds, and sliding into group chats with a simple "You HAVE to see this." It's fast, catchy, and engineered to be nearly impossible to ignore. Whether it's the latest celebrity drama, a wild conspiracy theory, or a 30-second video that's suddenly taking over the internet, the temptation to click is real—and the next thing you know, you've lost an hour diving into something you didn't even care about when you woke up.

But here's the thing: viral content isn't just accidentally captivating. It's carefully crafted to hook you. Platforms rely on your curiosity to keep you scrolling because the longer you stay, the more ads they can show you. The most successful viral content doesn't just entertain—it triggers psychological responses designed to override your impulse control. From provocative headlines that stir up emotion to cliffhanger videos that "promise" a payoff, every piece of viral media is engineered to hijack your attention.

Understanding why you're drawn to viral rabbit holes is the first step to resisting them. At the core is a powerful cognitive bias called the curiosity gap—the space between what you know and what you want to know. Viral content thrives on teasing that gap with headlines like "You'll NEVER believe what happened next!" or "This one secret will blow your mind." Your brain craves closure, and the only way to close the loop is to click. This is why even the most ridiculous or trivial content can feel irresistible—it preys on your brain's need to resolve uncertainty.

The algorithms behind your favorite platforms know this all too well. They're not just passive systems delivering content randomly—they actively learn what holds your attention and feed you more of it. If you click on one viral post about a celebrity breakup, the algorithm assumes you'll want similar content, creating a feedback loop where one click leads to another. And because these systems prioritize engagement over everything else, the most emotionally provocative content rises to the top. It's not just what you want to see—it's what will keep you hooked the longest.

To break free from this loop, you need to pause before you click—and that's harder than it sounds. Viral content is designed to override rational thinking by hitting your emotional buttons. Outrage, curiosity, and surprise are especially powerful triggers. When you see a post that makes you want to click immediately, stop for five seconds and ask yourself: "Do I actually care about this, or am I being manipulated?" This brief moment of reflection disrupts the automatic urge to dive deeper. Most viral content doesn't stand up to scrutiny—when you pause, you often realize it's not worth your time.

Another effective strategy is to practice intentional curiosity— the art of choosing what deserves your attention instead of letting algorithms decide. Viral rabbit holes often leave you feeling empty because they provide shallow, fleeting satisfaction. Instead of chasing whatever is trending, focus on content that genuinely aligns with your interests and values. You can train your brain to prioritize meaningful curiosity by setting a simple rule: If it doesn't improve your mood, expand your knowledge, or deepen your relationships, it's probably not worth your time.

But what about those times when the pull is too strong? Sometimes, no matter how mindful you try to be, the allure of a viral rabbit hole feels irresistible. When that happens, redirect the impulse without suppressing it entirely. Curiosity is natural—and fighting it head-on often backfires. Instead of forcing yourself to ignore every tempting headline, give your brain a better outlet. When you feel the urge to click on something trivial, switch to a more intentional curiosity activity—like reading a long-form article, watching a documentary, or diving into a topic you've always wanted to explore. You're still feeding your curiosity, but on your terms.

A crucial piece of resisting viral rabbit holes lies in understanding the emotional manipulation baked into them. Viral posts are designed to provoke intense feelings—whether that's anger, amusement, or shock—because strong emotional reactions increase engagement. Each time you click on something that stirs a powerful emotion, the algorithm registers it as a win and will serve you more of the same. It's a cycle that conditions you to keep reacting instead of reflecting.

When you encounter something emotionally charged, ask yourself: "Is this designed to inform me, or just to make me react?" By consciously labeling emotional triggers, you weaken their grip on your attention. You can also shift from reactive consumption to reflective engagement. Instead of immediately responding to every sensational headline or viral video, develop the habit of asking deeper questions. What's the source? What's the agenda? Why is this being promoted now? This type of mental framing empowers you to stay in control instead of being led by impulsive emotions.

And then there's FOMO—the fear of missing out. Viral content exploits the anxiety that everyone else knows something you don't. The subtle implication is that if you don't watch or read it right now, you'll be left out of the conversation. This taps into a basic human desire for social belonging. But here's the truth: most viral content is disposable. A week from now, no one will remember the trending meme or the latest internet scandal. Ask yourself: "Will this matter to me tomorrow? Next week? Next year?" If the answer is no, it's probably not worth your time.

It's also important to redefine what staying informed really means. In the age of viral media, there's a pervasive fear that if you don't click, you'll miss something important. But most viral content isn't about essential knowledge—it's about entertainment and profit. Instead of relying on whatever surfaces in your feed, curate trusted sources that deliver meaningful, well-rounded information. When you're proactive about where you get your news and entertainment, the algorithm loses its power to dictate your digital experience.

To protect your attention, it helps to design your digital environment intentionally. Small tweaks—like disabling autoplay, unsubscribing from clickbaity channels, or removing social media notifications—can make a huge difference. The goal isn't to eliminate curiosity but to channel it in ways that nourish rather than drain you. Try setting specific times for intentional browsing, so you engage with content mindfully instead of falling into endless scroll loops. You can also create "curiosity lists"— topics you genuinely care about—and dedicate time to explore those instead of whatever's trending.

And if you do fall into a viral rabbit hole? Be kind to yourself—then course-correct. We've all been there, emerging from a deep scroll wondering where the last hour went. Blaming yourself only reinforces the behavior loop through shame. Instead, treat it as a signal that your brain needed stimulation. Ask yourself: "What was I looking for when I clicked? Distraction? Connection? Entertainment?" By identifying the emotional need behind the scroll, you can find healthier ways to meet it next time.

At the end of the day, resisting viral rabbit holes isn't about shutting yourself off from the internet entirely—it's about reclaiming your right to choose. You deserve a digital life where your curiosity serves you, not the algorithm. By pausing to reflect, practicing intentional curiosity, and recognizing emotional triggers, you can break free from the viral trap and engage with content on your own terms.

The internet isn't going to slow down—but you can. And when you do, you'll realize that the most meaningful things aren't buried in the next viral sensation. They're already within your reach—if you choose to focus on what truly matters.

PART 5

# Building a Healthier
# Digital Future

# 33

# Living Slow in a Fast-Scroll World

THE INTERNET MOVES FAST—TOO FAST. Blink, and there's a new viral moment. Refresh, and your feed fills with updates that scream for your attention. In a world where everything is instant—news, entertainment, reactions—it's easy to feel like you're always chasing the next thing. But living in a constant state of digital urgency takes a toll. Your brain wasn't built for endless input, and over time, that rapid-fire consumption leads to burnout, scattered thinking, and a growing inability to just pause.

Slowing down doesn't mean disconnecting completely—it means choosing how and when to engage. It's about reclaiming your mental space from the relentless speed of the digital world and allowing yourself to move with intention. While the internet rewards speed, your mind thrives in slowness—where ideas can breathe, emotions can settle, and real focus can emerge. But in a culture obsessed with faster, better, more, how do you actually embrace slowness without feeling left behind?

At the heart of digital speed culture is a craving for **immediacy**—and this desire is no accident. Tech platforms are designed to deliver content as quickly and seamlessly as possible because the faster you consume, the longer you stay. Algorithms prioritize content that generates rapid engagement, and the more you interact, the more personalized (and addictive) your digital world becomes. But this breakneck pace isn't just shaping your habits—it's reshaping your **brain**. Studies show that constant digital stimulation weakens your ability to focus deeply, process information meaningfully, and tolerate stillness. It's not just that we consume faster—we expect everything to be fast, from answers to gratification.

Living slow in a fast-scroll world means deliberately resisting this culture of constant acceleration. It's about creating breathing room between digital inputs instead of racing from one dopamine hit to the next. When you slow down, you give your brain the chance to engage more deeply with what matters—whether that's savoring an article instead of skimming, sitting with a thought instead of reacting instantly, or allowing curiosity to unfold without rushing to the next click. And while that might sound idealistic in a world that never stops, it's also entirely possible with small, intentional shifts.

One of the most powerful ways to embrace slowness online is by **single-tasking**—doing one thing at a time, with your full attention. Multitasking is often worn like a badge of honor, but the truth is, your brain isn't designed to handle multiple streams of information simultaneously. What feels like multitasking is actually **task-switching**—a process that drains mental energy, increases cognitive fatigue, and reduces your ability to focus. Research shows that people who switch between tasks experience a **40% reduction in productivity** and take longer to regain focus.

When you single-task online, you resist the urge to bounce between tabs, apps, and notifications. It's choosing to read one article fully instead of opening five. It's watching a video without simultaneously scrolling through your feed. It's allowing yourself to be fully present in one digital moment instead of fragmenting your attention. And while it might feel uncomfortable at first— like your brain is itching for the next thing—this discomfort is a sign that you're retraining your mental muscles for **deep focus**.

One simple practice to cultivate single-tasking is the **15-minute rule**. When you start a digital activity—whether it's reading, watching, or creating—commit to staying with it for 15 minutes before switching to anything else. This small window helps your brain settle into a deeper state of focus while building resilience against distraction. Over time, these mindful pauses compound, strengthening your ability to stay present both online and offline.

Another key to living slow is learning to **tolerate boredom**—and this is harder than it sounds in a world where stimulation is always a tap away. Digital culture conditions us to view boredom as a problem to be solved immediately, but boredom is actually a **gateway to creativity and clarity**. When your mind isn't bombarded with constant input, it naturally begins to wander, make connections, and reflect on deeper thoughts.

Instead of filling every empty moment with digital noise, try leaving space for boredom to unfold. Resist the urge to check your phone in every spare second—whether you're waiting in line, sitting on the train, or winding down before bed. These micro-pauses might feel unproductive, but they give your brain the break it needs to process, reset, and generate fresh ideas. You're not wasting time—you're reclaiming mental bandwidth.

A slower digital life also means questioning the **urgency culture** baked into online spaces. Social media thrives on making everything feel immediate—respond now, react now, stay updated 24/7. But most things aren't as urgent as they seem. Breaking free from this cycle starts with asking yourself: **"Is this truly urgent, or is it just designed to feel urgent?"** Often, the pressure to respond instantly is an illusion created by platforms that benefit from your constant engagement.

Practice **delaying digital responses** when possible. If a message or notification isn't urgent, let it sit for an hour (or even a day) before responding. If you encounter emotionally charged content, wait before reacting. This intentional slowness disrupts the reflex to respond immediately, giving you time to process and engage from a grounded place. It also reinforces the idea that your time and attention aren't automatically available on demand—they're yours to manage.

To embrace slowness fully, it's also crucial to examine your **relationship with instant gratification**. Platforms are designed to deliver rewards fast—whether it's likes, comments, or content that triggers an emotional high. But this quick-reward cycle trains your brain to seek short-term pleasure over long-term fulfillment. Slowing down means rewiring this impulse by choosing **delayed gratification**—investing your attention in things that may not offer instant payoff but provide deeper, lasting value.

One simple way to shift this mindset is by curating a **slow content diet**. Instead of defaulting to whatever is most clickable or immediate, seek out content that takes time to engage with. Long-form essays, documentaries, reflective podcasts—these slower mediums encourage depth over speed. You're not just consuming—you're absorbing. And in a world that prioritizes quick hits, the ability to stay with something longer is a radical act of care for your mind.

At its core, living slow isn't about rejecting technology—it's about reclaiming **choice**. It's deciding where your attention goes, how quickly you move, and what pace feels right for your mental health. It's allowing yourself to exist beyond the algorithm's demands and finding freedom in moments of stillness.

And here's the truth: nothing important is lost by slowing down. The internet will keep moving at its relentless pace, but you don't have to follow. When you resist the pressure to always be faster, better, and more responsive, you make space for what truly matters—clarity, calm, and a life that feels like your own.

# 34

# Rediscovering Real Life

THERE S A CERTAIN MAGIC TO life that screens just can't replicate. The smell of the air after a rainstorm, the belly laughs during a spontaneous hangout, the quiet thrill of getting lost in a hobby—these moments have a texture that no filter or post can capture. And yet, in a world where the digital and physical blur, it's easy to forget how good real life can feel. Scrolling may keep you occupied, but living offline is where the real glow-up happens—deep joy, rich memories, and a sense of being truly present in your own story.

But let's be honest: the pull of the online world is strong. It's where conversations happen, where you share your wins, and where endless entertainment is just a tap away. Social media is designed to keep you hooked, feeding you an infinite stream of updates, memes, and viral moments. And while there's nothing inherently wrong with that, too much digital immersion can dull your ability to experience real life fully. When every quiet moment is filled with scrolling, you lose the capacity to be present—to savor the world as it unfolds around you.

The truth? Your brain craves offline experiences. Studies show that activities like being in nature, engaging in face-to-face conversation, and practicing hands-on hobbies activate parts of the brain linked to emotional regulation, creativity, and long-term memory. When you unplug from the constant buzz of digital life, you allow your nervous system to reset, reducing anxiety and improving your ability to focus. It's not about rejecting technology—it's about creating space for the kind of experiences that nourish you on a deeper level.

One of the most powerful shifts you can make is reclaiming your time from passive digital consumption and investing it in real-life activities that bring you joy. Think about the things you loved before screens took over—hobbies, interests, simple pleasures. When was the last time you lost yourself in a book for hours? Or spent an afternoon creating something with your hands? These moments aren't just "nice to have"—they're essential for mental clarity and emotional well-being.

Reconnecting with real-life joy starts by noticing how much of your time is spent consuming versus creating and experiencing. Consumption is easy—it's scrolling, watching, reacting. But creating? That's where the magic is. It could be as simple as cooking a new recipe, doodling in a notebook, or dancing around your room with zero regard for how it looks. The point isn't to be good at it—the point is to do it. Engaging in offline creativity rewires your brain for curiosity and presence, giving you a break from the endless loop of digital input.

For many, the biggest fear of unplugging is missing out. FOMO is real, and the internet is designed to amplify it. Every scroll shows you what others are doing—what you could be doing—creating a sense that life is happening somewhere else. But here's the catch: the more you chase online validation, the less rooted you feel in your actual life. The solution isn't to quit the internet entirely—it's to reframe what you value. Instead of chasing every update, prioritize the experiences that make you feel full—the ones that don't need an audience to matter.

One simple way to shift your perspective is by embracing JOMO—the joy of missing out. This isn't about withdrawing from the world: it's about recognizing that you don't need to be everywhere or know everything to live fully. JOMO means choosing activities that nourish you over ones that drain you. It's the quiet pleasure of spending a Saturday offline, immersed in things that ground you—without feeling the itch to document or share. The real glow-up isn't in being seen—it's in being present.

And while online connection has its place, there's something irreplaceable about in-person experiences. No amount of heart emojis can replicate the warmth of a friend's laugh. Physical presence triggers a cascade of feel-good chemicals—oxytocin, serotonin—that boost mood and deepen emotional bonds. In contrast, studies show that too much digital interaction can increase feelings of loneliness and disconnection, especially when it replaces face-to-face contact.

So, how do you start building a life where offline joy coexists with digital convenience? It begins with small, intentional choices. You don't need to disappear from the internet—but you do need to create boundaries that protect your real-life time. Start by carving out tech-free pockets during your day:

Morning magic: Begin your day without screens. Whether it's journaling, stretching, or simply sitting with your thoughts, these quiet moments set the tone for a calmer, more grounded day.

Offline oases: Designate spaces in your home where screens are off-limits—your bedroom, the dinner table, or a cozy reading nook. These tech-free zones become invitations to engage with the physical world.

Analog adventures: Schedule regular offline activities—go for a hike, take a pottery class, or visit a museum. These experiences create memories that stick, because your brain encodes them more deeply without digital distraction.

Another transformative practice? Digital sabbaths. Choose one day a week (or even a few hours) where you unplug fully. No scrolling, no notifications—just real life. It might feel weird at first—like you're missing something—but soon, you'll notice the opposite: a feeling of spaciousness, clarity, and a reconnection to the world around you.

And here's the thing—your offline glow-up doesn't mean rejecting the internet entirely. It means knowing when to engage and when to step back. It's the power of choice—choosing to savor a sunset instead of photographing it, to linger in a conversation instead of checking your phone, to live fully instead of curating a highlight reel.

When you prioritize real life, everything changes. The pressure to keep up fades. Your nervous system resets. You remember what it feels like to simply be. And in a world that constantly demands your attention, that kind of presence is a radical act of self-care.

The best memories? They don't live on your camera roll. They live in the moments when you forget to check your phone because real life is too good to miss. And that's the heart of the offline glow-up—it's not about what you lose by unplugging. It's about everything you gain.

# 35

# The Power of Digital Rest

IN A WORLD WHERE EVERY second can be filled with a notification, a meme, or a breaking news alert, the idea of doing nothing—even for a moment—feels almost radical. The digital age doesn't just steal your time; it hijacks your mental bandwidth, leaving little room for reflection or rest. Yet, research suggests that one of the most powerful tools for reclaiming your focus and emotional balance isn't a grand digital detox—it's something much simpler: **micro-breaks.** These small pauses, scattered throughout your day, create the mental breathing room your brain desperately needs in an always-on world.

Think of your mind as a browser with too many tabs open. Each notification, each scroll, and each new piece of content adds another tab. At first, your system can handle it. But over time, without a reset, the mental clutter slows your processing speed, drains your energy, and leaves you feeling mentally fried. Micro-breaks act like a "refresh" button—giving your brain a chance to clear the backlog and operate more efficiently.

Your brain wasn't designed to absorb the nonstop influx of information modern technology throws at it. Each time you switch tasks—say, from reading an article to checking a notification—you engage in "task-switching," a process that forces your brain to pause, reset, and refocus. Studies show that frequent task-switching can reduce cognitive efficiency by up to **40%**. Essentially, the more you hop between digital distractions, the harder it becomes to focus deeply on anything.

But here's the good news: **micro-breaks**—short pauses from screen time—reverse this cognitive drain. Research from the University of Illinois found that taking breaks as brief as **5-10 minutes** improves mental clarity, reduces fatigue, and restores focus. These breaks work because your brain thrives on cycles of activity and rest. When you interrupt the endless scroll with intentional pauses, you give your mind the space to reset and function optimally.

## Why Micro-Breaks Work (Even if They're Tiny)

You don't need a full-day tech detox to feel the benefits of digital rest. Even **short, intentional pauses**—as brief as a few minutes—disrupt the mental autopilot that screens induce. These breaks reduce mental fatigue by allowing your brain's default mode network (DMN) to activate. This is the brain region linked to creativity, self-reflection, and problem-solving—things that get buried under the constant flood of digital stimuli.

A fascinating study published in *Nature* found that even **brief cognitive breathers**—moments where you pause and disengage from active focus—improve memory retention and emotional regulation. When you step away from screens, your brain processes and consolidates information more effectively, turning fragmented experiences into meaningful insights.

In short: The less you push your brain without pause, the better it performs.

## Designing Micro-Breaks That Fit Your Life

The beauty of micro-breaks? You can seamlessly weave them into your daily routine without disrupting your flow. Here's how to make digital rest work for you:

- The 5-Minute Reset: Set aside five minutes every hour to disconnect. Put down your phone, step away from your screen, and give your brain a breather. Use this time to stretch, hydrate, or simply let your mind wander. These micro-pauses recalibrate your nervous system, reducing the mental fog caused by overstimulation.
- The 20-20-20 Rule: For every 20 minutes of screen time, look at something 20 feet away for at least 20 seconds. This simple habit eases digital eye strain while providing a mini-mental reset. It's a small shift that makes a big difference in how refreshed you feel by the end of the day.
- Tech-Free Transitions: Use life's natural pauses—waiting for your coffee, commuting, brushing your teeth—as opportunities for screen-free moments. These "in-between" times, often filled by mindless scrolling, become pockets of restorative rest when left uninterrupted.
- Sensory Micro-Breaks: Engage your senses during your pauses to ground yourself in the present. Smell fresh air, listen to birdsong, or feel the warmth of sunlight. This sensory engagement pulls you out of digital overstimulation and reconnects you to the physical world.

## The Power of Mental Space in a Hyper-Connected World

The irony of digital life is that the more connected you are online, the more disconnected you can feel from yourself. Constant input leaves no room for reflection, creativity, or emotional processing. Micro-breaks reintroduce mental spaciousness—the kind that fosters new ideas, emotional clarity, and a sense of calm.

Consider the last time you had a breakthrough idea. It probably didn't happen while doomscrolling Twitter. More likely, it arrived during a quiet moment—while taking a walk, washing the dishes, or daydreaming. That's because your brain does its best work when it has space to roam freely. Micro-breaks cultivate these fertile mental landscapes, giving your mind the room it needs to function at its best.

In a productivity-obsessed culture, the idea of pausing can feel counterintuitive—like you're wasting time. But the reality? Regular digital rest boosts both creativity and productivity. By stepping back, even briefly, you allow your mind to recover and work smarter, not harder.

Athletes understand the importance of rest days for physical recovery—your brain operates the same way. Without breaks, you burn out. With them, you thrive. And the best part? Micro-breaks don't require dramatic lifestyle changes—they fit into the rhythm of your day.

The most important shift you can make is seeing digital rest as essential, not optional. Here are a few final ways to make it part of your daily life:

- Pre-schedule your pauses: Set reminders to take brief screen-free breaks. Treat them like appointments with your mental well-being.

- Honor the first and last 10 minutes of your day: Start and end your day without screens. Give yourself the gift of quiet space before the digital world rushes in.

- Celebrate the small pauses: Even a single deep breath between tasks counts. Every pause is a step toward reclaiming your mental clarity.

When you prioritize micro-breaks, you disrupt the endless loop of input and give yourself the gift of presence. It's not about rejecting technology—it's about using it consciously without letting it drain your mental reserves.

In a world that glorifies being constantly "on," stepping back— even briefly—is an act of quiet rebellion. It's a reminder that your mind is worth protecting. And in those small, deliberate pauses? That's where the real magic happens.

# 36

# Unplugging without Missing Out

EVERY MOMENT IS A POTENTIAL post, the fear of missing out—
FOMO—has evolved from a fleeting feeling to a near-constant
hum in the background of our digital lives. It's not just the
worry that you're missing a party or an event; it's the sense that
somewhere, someone is living a shinier, more exciting version of
life while you're stuck in the ordinary. Social media amplifies this
anxiety, curating highlight reels that blur the line between reality
and performance. And yet, for all its promises of connection,
being perpetually plugged in can leave you feeling more isolated
and out of sync with your actual life.

The idea of unplugging sounds simple enough—log off, step
away, reclaim your time. But in practice, the fear creeps in. What if
you miss something important? What if everyone else is bonding
over a meme or a trending conversation you're not part of? That
tug of FOMO isn't just about curiosity—it's tied to a deeper human
need to belong. Yet the paradox is clear: the more you chase
digital connection, the more you risk losing real-life presence.

Unplugging without feeling left out isn't about abandoning
the online world altogether. It's about redefining how you engage
with it—on your terms. It means shifting from a reactive, fear-
driven mindset to a more intentional, joyful approach. Because
behind the polished perfection and endless updates, what most

people really crave isn't another scroll through their feed—it's a sense of meaning and connection that can't be captured in pixels.

## The FOMO Illusion: Why It's Never the Whole Story

At its core, FOMO is fueled by perception rather than reality. When you see a friend's beach vacation or a group selfie from a night out, you're not just observing the moment—you're filling in the gaps. The brain has a tendency to **romanticize the unknown**, assuming that whatever is happening without you must be better, cooler, or more fulfilling. What you don't see are the mundane in-between moments—the overpriced cocktails, the awkward silences, the exhaustion that isn't Instagram-worthy.

Social media thrives on this carefully crafted illusion. Every platform is designed to keep you hooked by feeding that gnawing sense that something more exciting is always happening elsewhere. But the reality? Most people aren't living the dazzling, cinematic lives their profiles suggest. Studies show that frequent social media users report higher levels of loneliness and anxiety precisely because the comparison trap is so relentless. When your baseline for "normal" is filtered through curated content, your everyday life starts to feel impossibly dull by contrast.

But here's the truth: You're not missing as much as you think. And the experiences that matter most—the deep conversations, the quiet joys, the sense of belonging—rarely make it to the highlight reel. Real life happens in the gaps between posts, in the messy, unscripted moments that social media can't fully capture.

## The Joy of Missing Out: Embracing What Matters

If FOMO is fueled by scarcity—the idea that you're missing limited-time experiences—then **JOMO**, the joy of missing out, is its antidote. JOMO flips the narrative, reframing disconnection not as deprivation, but as a conscious choice to prioritize what truly nourishes you. It's about recognizing that your attention is a finite resource, and you get to decide where it goes.

Embracing JOMO isn't about becoming a digital recluse. It's about reclaiming your time and mental energy for things that actually make you feel whole. Instead of chasing every notification or event, you cultivate a mindset that values **depth over breadth**—choosing fewer, richer experiences over a constant stream of superficial ones.

This shift requires a bit of unlearning. We've been conditioned to see availability as a virtue—to be always on, always reachable. But real connection isn't measured by the number of conversations you have; it's measured by the quality of the ones that matter. When you step back from the noise, you make room for the relationships and activities that bring genuine fulfillment.

## Redefining Connection: Quality over Constant Access

One of the biggest myths about unplugging is that it means cutting yourself off from others. In reality, being hyper-connected often dilutes the quality of your relationships. When you're juggling a dozen group chats and scrolling through endless updates, it's easy to mistake **proximity** for **closeness**. But being digitally present doesn't automatically translate to emotional intimacy.

Unplugging gives you the opportunity to be more **selective** and **intentional** with your connections. It means choosing to engage with people in ways that feel meaningful rather than performative. You don't have to be the first to react to every post or stay in the loop with every online conversation to maintain your relationships. In fact, stepping back can deepen your connections by allowing you to show up more fully when it truly matters.

Consider this: Who do you actually want to invest your time and energy in? Whose presence feels nourishing rather than draining? By curating your social interactions—both online and offline—you create space for relationships that feel mutual, supportive, and aligned with your values.

## Setting Boundaries Without the Guilt

The fear of missing out often disguises a deeper anxiety—the worry that by stepping back, you'll somehow become irrelevant or invisible. But maintaining a constant online presence isn't the same as being seen in a meaningful way. True connection doesn't require constant visibility; it requires intentional presence.

Setting digital boundaries is an act of self-respect, not disconnection. It's about recognizing your limits and protecting your mental and emotional well-being. You can stay engaged without being perpetually available. And you can say no to the endless scroll without saying no to the people who matter.

Here are a few ways to set boundaries while staying connected:

- Communicate your limits: Let people know when you're taking a step back from certain platforms or reducing your availability. Most people will respect your boundaries when they understand your intention.
- Prioritize in-person connection: Whenever possible, choose face-to-face interactions over digital ones. These moments foster deeper bonds and reduce the sense of superficial engagement.
- Be intentional with your time: Schedule specific windows for checking in online rather than defaulting to constant access. This helps you stay connected while preserving time for offline life.

## The Freedom of Choosing What Matters

At the heart of unplugging without missing out is a profound truth: **You get to choose what matters to you.** When you stop chasing every digital distraction, you reclaim the freedom to invest in experiences that bring lasting joy. The world won't fall apart if you miss a trending meme or skip an online debate. But the moments you spend fully present—laughing with friends, immersing yourself in a passion project, savoring quiet solitude— these are the moments that stay with you.

Unplugging isn't about rejecting the digital world entirely. It's about stepping into a life where your attention is no longer held hostage by FOMO. Instead of being pulled in every direction, you become the curator of your own experiences. You learn to trust that what's meant for you won't pass you by—and in that trust, you find a new kind of freedom.

When you unplug with intention, you discover that real life—the messy, beautiful, imperfect reality—is far richer than anything a screen can deliver. And perhaps the greatest joy of all is realizing that you were never really missing out—you were simply making room for what truly matters.

# 37

# From Consumer to Creator

EVERY SCROLL, CLICK, AND LIKE on the internet feeds a system designed to keep you consuming. It's easy to lose hours watching other people's lives unfold—snacking on content that's polished, curated, and often far from reality. In this never-ending stream of videos, photos, and hot takes, the line between observer and participant blurs. You're watching, but are you really engaging? The algorithms want you passive—quietly absorbing endless content without questioning how it shapes your thoughts, habits, and self-image. But there's another way to exist online—one where you aren't just a consumer but a creator, reclaiming your digital space on your terms.

Shifting from consumption to creation isn't just about posting more. It's about ownership—choosing how you engage with the digital world rather than letting it shape you. When you move from mindless scrolling to intentional expression, something shifts. You become an active participant instead of a bystander. Your ideas, experiences, and creativity stop being passive reactions and become contributions that reflect who you are and what you care about. And in a world where it's easier than ever to consume, creating gives you something that endless scrolling never can—a sense of agency.

## The Consumption Trap: How Passive Habits Shape Your Mind

It's no accident that modern digital platforms are built to encourage consumption. Every detail—endless feeds, autoplay, infinite scroll—is engineered to keep you in a passive state. The longer you stay, the more data you generate, and the more profitable you become. But this constant consumption doesn't just drain your time—it shapes how you think, what you value, and even how you see yourself.

When you consume without intention, you absorb more than just content. You internalize subtle messages about what's valuable, desirable, and worthy of attention. You start comparing your life to curated highlights. You lose time to content that doesn't reflect your priorities or add to your growth. And maybe without realizing it, you start living more reactively—chasing trends instead of shaping your own voice.

Passive consumption also limits creativity. Research shows that when the brain is constantly bombarded by external stimuli, it has fewer opportunities to engage in the deep thought processes that fuel creativity and innovation. In other words, the more you consume, the harder it becomes to create. Constant input drowns out your own ideas, leaving little room for reflection, originality, or self-expression.

## The Empowerment of Creating over Consuming

Becoming a creator in the digital age isn't just about sharing content—it's about reclaiming your mental space and redefining your relationship with technology. When you create instead of consume, you shift from being shaped by the algorithm to shaping your own narrative.

This shift is powerful because creation is inherently active—it demands thought, engagement, and presence. Whether you're writing, making art, recording a podcast, or simply sharing your perspective, creation pushes you to contribute rather than just absorb. And unlike the fleeting satisfaction of mindless scrolling, the act of creating taps into something deeper—a sense of purpose and meaning.

Creating also builds psychological resilience. When you express yourself intentionally, you begin to value your unique perspective over external validation. Instead of chasing likes or follows, you prioritize work that feels authentic. And this internal focus gives you more control over your emotional experience online. Rather than being at the mercy of how others react, you find satisfaction in the process of making itself.

And here's the thing—you don't need to be an influencer or a professional artist to be a creator. You just need to start. Whether you're journaling privately, sharing your thoughts on a niche topic, or documenting your hobbies, what matters isn't scale—it's intention. It's the choice to engage with technology on your own terms, creating content that reflects your values, interests, and identity.

## Creating Content That Reflects Who You Are

In a digital world obsessed with virality and trends, it's easy to feel like what you create has to fit a mold. But real, meaningful creation doesn't come from chasing the latest trend—it comes from expressing what genuinely resonates with you. When you create content that reflects your values and identity, you reclaim the narrative about who you are and what you stand for.

Start by asking yourself: What do I care about? What stories or ideas feel worth sharing? Your digital presence doesn't need to be a highlight reel or a performance. It can be a reflection of your real life—the messy, beautiful, evolving parts that algorithms can't capture. Whether it's through writing, video, art, or conversation, the medium doesn't matter as much as the message. What counts is that it's yours.

There's also freedom in creating without the pressure to perform. You don't need a massive audience to make your voice matter. Some of the most powerful forms of digital creation are small-scale—writing a thoughtful newsletter, making a playlist that reflects your mood, sharing ideas with a small community. These acts of creation are about **connection** rather than clout. They remind you that your voice has value beyond likes or shares.

## Finding Fulfillment through Intentional Contribution

When you shift from consuming to creating, you're not just taking back your time—you're cultivating **fulfillment**. Passive consumption offers quick hits of dopamine, but those fleeting rewards fade fast. Creation, on the other hand, taps into something more enduring—the sense that your contributions matter.

This kind of fulfillment comes from a deeper place. It's the satisfaction of seeing your ideas take form, of building something that didn't exist before. It's the pride in knowing that you're not just reacting to the digital world—you're shaping it in ways that align with your values.

Intentional contribution also fosters a **sense of community**. When you create from a place of authenticity, you attract people who resonate with your message. These connections are richer and more meaningful than the surface-level engagement of endless scrolling. They remind you that your voice isn't just noise—it's a part of a larger conversation.

If you're ready to take back control and start creating, the shift doesn't have to be dramatic. Small, intentional changes can help you break free from passive habits and reclaim your digital space.

1. Limit Passive Consumption – Set boundaries around when and how you engage with content. Be mindful of how much time you spend consuming versus creating.

2. Create Before You Consume – Each day, prioritize making something—whether it's a journal entry, a sketch, or a thoughtful post—before you dive into other people's content.

3. Share What Feels Authentic – Focus on expressing ideas and experiences that reflect who you are, rather than chasing trends or external approval.

4. Engage with Purpose – Use your digital platforms intentionally. Seek out communities and conversations that align with your values and interests.

At its core, moving from consumer to creator is about **choice**. It's the decision to take back control of your digital experience, to engage with intention, and to express yourself in ways that matter. And in a world designed to keep you scrolling, that choice is a radical act of self-empowerment.

When you stop consuming mindlessly and start creating with purpose, you change the game. You stop being a passive player in someone else's narrative and become the author of your own. And that's a power no algorithm can take away.

# 38

# Staying Smart in the Age of AI Manipulation

EVERY TIME YOU OPEN YOUR phone, artificial intelligence is quietly working behind the scenes—curating, filtering, and deciding what you see next. From the articles you read to the products you buy, algorithms are shaping your reality in ways that feel seamless but are anything but neutral. The era of AI-driven content isn't coming—it's already here, and it's transforming how we perceive information, form opinions, and even understand ourselves. In a world where machines learn your preferences better than you know them, staying sharp isn't just a skill—it's a survival strategy.

At its core, AI manipulation isn't about flashy robots or dystopian futures. It's subtle, personalized, and often invisible. Every click, like, and share feeds these systems more data—training them to deliver content that captures your attention and keeps you scrolling. And while personalized feeds might seem convenient, they also create echo chambers, nudge your decisions, and quietly shape your worldview. Understanding how AI influences you isn't about paranoia—it's about maintaining agency in a digital ecosystem that profits from your passivity.

## How AI Shapes What You See

AI doesn't just deliver random content—it delivers *your* content. Every digital interaction leaves behind data points that algorithms analyze and use to refine what you encounter next. Over time, this creates a hyper-personalized feed that reflects your habits, interests, and even your emotional triggers. This process—called algorithmic curation—is designed to maximize engagement, not accuracy or objectivity.

Consider your social media timeline. You aren't seeing a neutral, chronological list of posts. Instead, AI prioritizes content that it predicts will hold your attention the longest. It amplifies posts that evoke strong emotional reactions—outrage, joy, or even fear—because those feelings keep you hooked. Meanwhile, content that doesn't align with your previous clicks quietly fades from view, reinforcing your existing beliefs while shielding you from alternative perspectives.

This curated reality has a profound effect on how you think and behave. Research shows that people exposed only to algorithmically filtered news are more likely to develop polarized opinions. And it's not just politics—AI-driven feeds shape everything from how you perceive beauty standards to what you consider normal in relationships. When you only see a slice of reality tailored to your preferences, it's easy to mistake that slice for the whole picture.

## The Subtle Art of Persuasion: How AI Nudges Your Decisions

AI doesn't just reflect your choices—it shapes them. From product recommendations to search engine results, algorithms are constantly nudging you toward certain decisions. This phenomenon, known as algorithmic persuasion, is subtle but powerful. Instead of forcing you to make a choice, AI steers you toward specific outcomes by controlling the options you see.

Take online shopping. Platforms don't just show you random items—they show you products tailored to your browsing history, previous purchases, and even the time of day you're shopping. Studies show that personalized recommendations increase the likelihood of purchase by up to 37%—not because the products are better, but because they feel more relevant.

And the nudging doesn't stop there. Streaming services curate playlists designed to keep you binge-watching. News feeds prioritize stories that align with your worldview, reinforcing your biases. Even dating apps use AI to suggest matches based on behavioral data—shaping who you meet and how you connect. The longer you engage, the more predictive the system becomes, making it harder to recognize how much of your experience is being engineered.

The danger lies in how invisible these nudges are. Unlike traditional advertising, where persuasion is obvious, AI works behind the scenes—shaping your decisions while maintaining the illusion of free choice. And because the manipulation feels subtle, it's easy to dismiss the influence it has over your thoughts, preferences, and even identity.

## Staying Critical: How to Recognize AI's Influence

In an era where AI touches almost every aspect of your digital life, developing algorithmic awareness is crucial. This means recognizing when your choices are being influenced—and questioning the systems shaping your reality.

Start by paying attention to patterns. Notice how your feed changes based on your behavior. What types of content get amplified? Which perspectives are missing? The next time you're drawn to a viral post, ask yourself: Is this content valuable, or is it just engineered to hold my attention? Developing this reflexive awareness helps you separate what's real from what's being fed to you.

Another key strategy is to disrupt the algorithm. AI thrives on predictability—when you engage in repetitive behaviors, it refines its recommendations. By breaking your patterns—following new voices, reading diverse perspectives, and searching for content outside your usual preferences—you introduce randomness into the system. This disrupts the feedback loop and broadens the range of information you encounter.

And don't underestimate the power of pausing. Algorithms are optimized for speed—they rely on your instant reactions to shape future suggestions. By slowing down and questioning your impulses, you reclaim control. Before clicking on a headline or engaging with emotionally charged content, pause and ask: Is this true? Is this useful? Do I actually care? This micro-delay helps you resist algorithmic manipulation and make intentional choices.

## Tools to Stay Sharp in an AI-Dr ven World

Fortunately, you're not powerless against algorithmic influence. With the right tools and habits, you can navigate the digital landscape **on your terms**—engaging with technology without letting it shape you.

Use Privacy Tools – AI relies on data to personalize your experience. Limit what you share by using privacy-focused search engines (like DuckDuckGo), installing tracker blockers, and adjusting your platform privacy settings.

Diversify Your Information Sources – Break free from algorithmic bubbles by seeking information from independent sources. Subscribe to newsletters from credible journalists, explore open-access platforms, and actively seek out voices outside your typical circle.

Audit Your Digital Diet – Regularly assess the content you consume. Are your feeds enriching your understanding, or are they reinforcing narrow viewpoints? Curate your online experience by following accounts that challenge your assumptions.

Control Your Recommendations – Many platforms allow you to reset or customize their algorithms. Take advantage of these features—clear your watch history, disable personalized ads, and manually curate your content.

Practice Digital Minimalism – The less data you feed the algorithm, the less it can manipulate you. Limit mindless scrolling by setting screen-time boundaries, creating tech-free zones, and engaging with purpose rather than passivity.

Ultimately, staying smart in the age of AI manipulation is about reclaiming your agency. It's recognizing that while algorithms shape your experience, they don't control your choices—unless you let them. By staying aware, questioning narratives, and engaging intentionally, you can exist in the digital age without becoming its product.

In a world where AI is constantly learning you, the real power lies in knowing yourself. The more you question, the less you're controlled. And that awareness is your strongest defense against a system designed to keep you scrolling.

# 39

# Owning Your Attention

THE WHOLE WORLD IS FIGHTING for your attention—notifications, viral trends, endless feeds—the real flex is owning it. Your attention is more than a fleeting moment; it's your most valuable resource. It shapes how you spend your time, what you prioritize, and ultimately, the kind of life you build. And yet, the modern digital ecosystem is designed to hijack it. Every ping and algorithm is engineered to pull you away from your own intentions, turning your focus into a commodity that platforms monetize. The question is: who's really in control?

Owning your attention isn't just about turning off notifications or deleting apps—it's a radical act of self-empowerment. It's the decision to direct your energy toward what matters instead of being at the mercy of digital distractions. It's the shift from passive consumer to active participant, from being led by the algorithm to leading your own experience. And in a culture that profits from your distraction, reclaiming your focus is nothing short of revolutionary.

## The Currency of Attention

Every time you click, scroll, or linger on a post, you're feeding an economic machine. Attention isn't just abstract—it's a $500 billion industry where your focus is the product. Social media platforms, news outlets, streaming services—they all compete for your time because your engagement translates to revenue. The longer you stay, the more they profit. And they know exactly how to keep you hooked.

The science behind attention capture is no accident. Platforms exploit the brain's reward system, delivering unpredictable dopamine hits through notifications, likes, and endless content loops. This "variable reward system" keeps you chasing the next hit—scrolling without realizing how much time has slipped away. It's the same psychological mechanism behind slot machines, but instead of a casino, your entire digital world becomes a game designed to keep you playing.

And the cost isn't just wasted time. Fragmented attention drains your mental energy and diminishes your ability to focus deeply. Studies show that constant digital interruptions impair working memory, increase stress, and reduce overall cognitive capacity. When your attention is scattered across endless digital noise, it becomes harder to be present—both online and in real life.

## Reclaiming Your Time as a Power Move

When you start treating your attention as something precious— something you actively choose how to spend—the dynamic shifts. Instead of being at the mercy of algorithms, you begin reclaiming your time as an act of autonomy. And nothing feels more powerful than realizing you don't have to be available to everything, all the time.

The first step is recognizing that attention is finite. You wake up every day with a limited supply, and every digital distraction consumes a portion of it. Once it's spent, it's gone. Imagine your attention as a bank account—every unnecessary scroll or endless thread drains that balance. Owning your attention means choosing how to invest it wisely.

It also means getting intentional about where your focus goes. Instead of defaulting to mindless consumption, you start asking: Is this worth my time? Does this align with what matters to me? It's not about cutting off the digital world entirely—it's about curating your experience in a way that serves you, not the algorithm.

## Protecting Your Mental Space Like It's Sacred

Once you reclaim your attention, the next step is defending it fiercely. This isn't about rigid productivity hacks—it's about creating boundaries that honor your mental space. Because when your attention is constantly divided, you lose the ability to engage deeply with anything. And deep engagement—the kind where you lose track of time because you're so immersed—is where meaning is built.

One of the most underrated power moves is designing attention rituals—simple habits that anchor you back to intentional focus. Whether it's starting your day offline, taking mindful breaks, or setting "no-scroll zones," these rituals act as buffers against the digital pull. It's about creating spaces where your mind can breathe without being constantly overstimulated.

But beyond habits, owning your attention is about permission—the permission to step back, to disengage, to prioritize your mental clarity. It's realizing you don't owe the internet your constant presence. You're allowed to disappear from the noise without explanation. You're allowed to take up space in your own life without being digitally available 24/7.

## Attention Is Agency

The ultimate power in owning your attention is realizing it shapes your reality. What you focus on determines how you experience the world. Let your attention be hijacked by outrage cycles and superficial content, and that's what colors your perception. Direct your attention toward meaning, growth, and relationships, and your world reflects that richness.

And here's the truth: when you own your attention, you own the narrative. You stop being a passive player in someone else's game and start defining your own. You get to decide what stories you consume, what voices you amplify, and how you engage with the digital world. No algorithm gets to dictate what matters to you—unless you let it.

Owning your attention isn't about perfection. You're going to get pulled in sometimes—it's human. But it's the act of returning— again and again—to what matters most. It's refusing to let your focus be scattered across a thousand meaningless distractions. It's recognizing that your time, your energy, and your mental space are yours to protect.

In a world that thrives on your distraction, reclaiming your attention is a rebellion. And the most empowering realization of all? You always have the power to take it back.

# 40

# Building a Future You Control

DIGITAL LANDSCAPES SHIFT BY THE second, the ultimate power move is designing a future where your brain—and your choices—stay firmly in your hands. Technology isn't slowing down. If anything, it's evolving faster than ever, with algorithms becoming sharper, AI growing smarter, and the digital pull intensifying daily. But here's the twist: no matter how advanced tech becomes, your mind is still the command center. The question isn't whether the digital world will change—it's whether you'll let it change you without your permission.

Owning your digital future isn't about fear or resistance. It's about agency—deciding how technology fits into your life instead of being molded by it. When you start making intentional decisions about how, when, and why you engage with the digital sphere, you reclaim the power to shape your reality. Your brain, your rules. And in a culture that thrives on keeping you plugged in and passive, choosing conscious tech use isn't just a lifestyle shift—it's an act of self-liberation.

Let's be honest: the online world isn't going anywhere. Social platforms will evolve, content will get even more immersive, and new forms of engagement will emerge. Avoiding it altogether? Unrealistic. But you're not powerless against it. The real magic lies in designing a digital ecosystem that works *for* you—not against you.

It starts by asking: What do I want my relationship with technology to look like? This isn't about vague ideas of balance; it's about creating a digital life that aligns with your core values. Is your goal to stay informed without drowning in news cycles? To connect with friends without feeling enslaved by constant notifications? To use technology as a tool—not a trap? Your answers shape the blueprint for a future where you stay in charge.

Think of your digital habits like a curated playlist. Just as you'd remove songs you don't vibe with, you have the power to cut out platforms, content, and habits that drain you. Unfollow accounts that make you feel less-than. Limit apps that hijack your attention. Prioritize tools that genuinely enhance your life—whether that's a meditation app, a journaling space, or a podcast that feeds your mind. This isn't about deprivation. It's about intention—letting your digital environment reflect the life you actually want.

## Future-Proofing Your Brain against Tech Manipulation

The truth is, tech manipulation is only getting more sophisticated. With AI algorithms fine-tuning your every click and emerging technologies tracking everything from eye movements to emotional responses, passivity isn't an option. If you want to stay ahead, you need to future-proof your brain against these invisible forces.

One of the most powerful ways to do this? Build mental friction. In a digital landscape designed for seamless consumption, creating small pauses between stimulus and response rewires your brain for autonomy. Before you tap on a headline or dive into a trending topic, stop and ask: Is this worth my attention? Is this serving me or just serving the algorithm?

These micro-pauses disrupt the autopilot loop tech thrives on.

They give you time to reclaim your focus before it's snatched away. Over time, these intentional breaks strengthen your brain's ability to resist manipulation. The more you question the narrative, the harder it becomes for technology to mold your thoughts without your consent.

And here's a secret: curiosity is your greatest weapon. Instead of accepting digital information at face value, develop a habit of critical inquiry. Who benefits from this content? What emotions is it trying to provoke? Is this information expanding my perspective—or narrowing it? When you cultivate a questioning mindset, you become harder to manipulate because you stop accepting digital realities as truth without investigation.

## Building Long-Term Habits for Conscious Tech Use

Short-term digital detoxes are cute—but the real flex is sustainable, long-term change. Owning your brain means developing habits that create lasting autonomy, not just temporary relief. And while that sounds big, it starts with small, daily practices that reinforce your agency.

Start by defining non-negotiable boundaries—personal rules that protect your mental space. Maybe that's maintaining tech-free mornings to give your brain a buffer before diving into the digital flood. Or perhaps it's setting screen-free zones during meals to anchor yourself in real-world connection. These boundaries aren't restrictions—they're tools for empowerment, giving you the freedom to engage on your terms.

Another game-changer? Practice deliberate consumption. Instead of passively absorbing whatever the algorithm throws your way, curate your digital diet. Follow creators who inspire and educate. Seek out content that challenges your worldview. Be intentional about what you allow into your mental ecosystem—

because what you consume shapes how you think.

Finally, prioritize digital rest. Your brain wasn't built for 24/7 input, and constant stimulation diminishes its capacity to think deeply and creatively. Schedule regular breaks where you unplug completely—whether that's a weekend offline, a monthly "scroll fast," or daily moments of stillness. These pauses aren't indulgent; they're essential for protecting your cognitive clarity in an always-on world.

At the heart of all this is a simple truth: Your brain is yours. No algorithm, no platform, no viral trend gets to dictate how you think, feel, or spend your time—unless you let it. Owning your attention means recognizing that you are the gatekeeper. And once you fully embrace that power, you become impossible to control.

The future of technology is uncertain, but your ability to choose will always be certain. You get to decide what role tech plays in your life. You get to set the rules. And that agency? It's the ultimate form of freedom.

So, as the digital world keeps evolving, let this be your guiding mantra: My brain, my rules. Because when you own your attention, you own your reality—and no algorithm can take that from you.